Report of the Regional Director
on the work of WHO in the European Region
in 2012–2013

REALIZING OUR VISION

The World Health Organization was established in 1948 as the specialized agency of the United Nations serving as the directing and coordinating authority for international health matters and public health. One of WHO's constitutional functions is to provide objective and reliable information and advice in the field of human health. It fulfils this responsibility in part through its publications programmes, seeking to help countries make policies that benefit public health and address their most pressing public health concerns.

The WHO Regional Office for Europe is one of six regional offices throughout the world, each with its own programme geared to the particular health problems of the countries it serves. The European Region embraces nearly 900 million people living in an area stretching from the Arctic Ocean in the north and the Mediterranean Sea in the south and from the Atlantic Ocean in the west to the Pacific Ocean in the east. The European programme of WHO supports all countries in the Region in developing and sustaining their own health policies, systems and programmes; preventing and overcoming threats to health; preparing for future health challenges; and advocating and implementing public health activities.

To ensure the widest possible availability of authoritative information and guidance on health matters, WHO secures broad international distribution of its publications and encourages their translation and adaptation. By helping to promote and protect health and prevent and control disease, WHO's books contribute to achieving the Organization's principal objective – the attainment by all people of the highest possible level of health.

Report of the Regional Director on the work of WHO in the European Region in 2012–2013

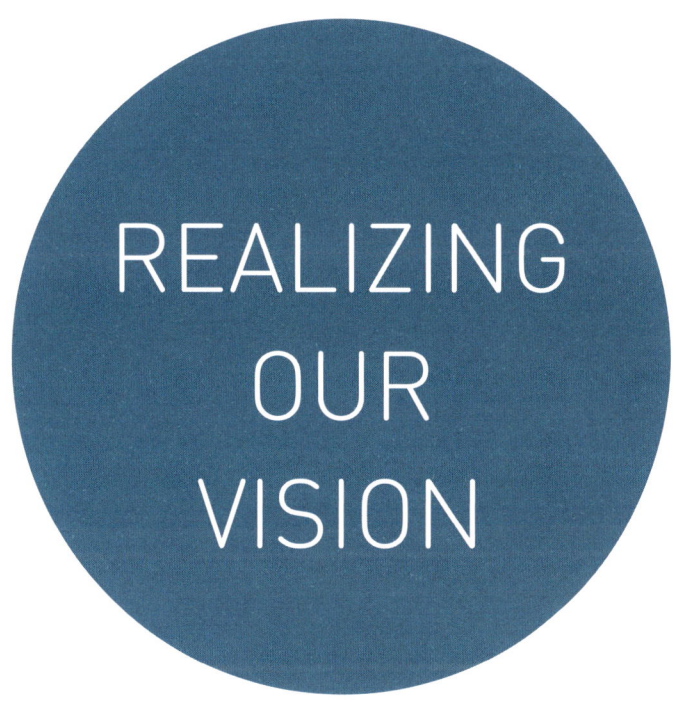

REALIZING OUR VISION

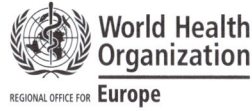

WHO Library Cataloguing-in-Publication Data

Realizing our vision: report of the Regional Director on the work of WHO in the European Region in 2012–2013.

1.Regional health planning. 2.World Health Organization. 3.Europe I.World Health Organization. Regional Office for Europe.

ISBN 978 92 890 5011 1 (print)   (NLM classification: WA 540)
ISBN 978 92 890 5017 3 (e-book)

ISBN 978 92 890 5011 1

Address requests about publications of the WHO Regional Office for Europe to:

    Publications
    WHO Regional Office for Europe
    UN City, Marmorvej 51
    DK-2100 Copenhagen Ø, Denmark

Alternatively, complete an online request form for documentation, health information, or for permission to quote or translate, on the Regional Office website (http://www.euro.who.int/pubrequest).

© **World Health Organization 2014**

All rights reserved. The Regional Office for Europe of the World Health Organization welcomes requests for permission to reproduce or translate its publications, in part or in full.

The designations employed and the presentation of the material in this publication do not imply the expression of any opinion whatsoever on the part of the World Health Organization concerning the legal status of any country, territory, city or area or of its authorities, or concerning the delimitation of its frontiers or boundaries. Dotted lines on maps represent approximate border lines for which there may not yet be full agreement.

The mention of specific companies or of certain manufacturers' products does not imply that they are endorsed or recommended by the World Health Organization in preference to others of a similar nature that are not mentioned. Errors and omissions excepted, the names of proprietary products are distinguished by initial capital letters.

All reasonable precautions have been taken by the World Health Organization to verify the information contained in this publication. However, the published material is being distributed without warranty of any kind, either express or implied. The responsibility for the interpretation and use of the material lies with the reader. In no event shall the World Health Organization be liable for damages arising from its use. The views expressed by authors, editors, or expert groups do not necessarily represent the decisions or the stated policy of the World Health Organization.

CONTENTS

Acronyms vii

Introduction: pursuing better health for Europe .. 1
Priorities and challenges 2

1. Tackling Europe's health challenges and priorities 3
Health 2020: the European policy for health and well-being 3
    Development and adoption 3
    Evidence base 4
    Implementation 5
    Targets and indicators: measuring health and well-being 7
Other work for equity and health development 8
    Vulnerable social groups 8
    MDGs and the post-2015 development agenda 9

2. Strengthening health systems 12
Action plan to rejuvenate public health 12
Comprehensive responses from health systems 13
    Supporting health system reforms in countries 15
    Working for the financial sustainability and resilience of health systems 16
    Training to build capacity 17
    Seeking a skilled and sustainable health workforce 18
Evidence and information for policy-making 19

3. NCDs and promoting health throughout life .. 22
Supporting comprehensive action 22
Promoting healthy behaviour 24
    Harmful alcohol use 24
    Tobacco control 24
    Nutrition and physical activity 25

    Mental health 27
    Violence and injury prevention 27
Promoting health throughout the life-course 28
    Maternal, child and adolescent health and well-being 28
    Healthy ageing 29

4. Communicable diseases 30
Implementing action plans 30
    M/XDR-TB 30
    HIV/AIDS 30
    Antibiotic resistance 31
Eliminating diseases 32
    Polio 32
    Malaria 33
    Measles and rubella 33
Promoting immunization 34
Re-emerging vector-borne and parasitic diseases .. 35

5. Preparedness, surveillance and response 36
Preparedness for emergencies and disasters 36
    International Health Regulations 36
    Preparedness 37
Surveillance 38
Responses to emergencies and disasters 38

6. European environment and health process 40
Governance 40
Technical work 41

7. Governance, partnerships and communication 43
Stronger governance in line with WHO reform 43
    Programmatic reform 43
    Governance reform 45
    Managerial reform 46

Financial overview 47
Deepening partnerships 48
Intensified collaboration with Member States 49
Strategic communications 50

References 51

Annex: Implementation of the programme budget for 2012–2013 66

ACRONYMS

Technical terms

CCSs	country cooperation strategies
CEHAPIS	climate, environment and health action plan and information system (WHO project)
CVD	cardiovascular diseases
DALY	disability-adjusted life-year
FCTC	WHO Framework Convention on Tobacco Control
GDO	geographically dispersed office (of the WHO Regional Office for Europe)
GPW	Twelfth General Programme of Work for 2014–2019
HBSC	Health Behaviour in School-aged Children (study)
IHR	International Health Regulations
MDGs	Millennium Development Goals
MERS-CoV	Middle East respiratory syndrome coronavirus
M/XDR-TB	multidrug- and extensively drug-resistant tuberculosis
NCDs	noncommunicable diseases
PACT	Programme of Action for Cancer Therapy
PHAME	Public Health Aspects of Migration in Europe (WHO project)
polio	poliomyelitis
SMART	specific, measurable, achievable, relevant and timely (targets)
TB	tuberculosis

Organizations, networks and other entities

ASPHER	Association of Schools of Public Health in the European Region
BMA	British Medical Association
CAESAR	Central Asia and Eastern European Surveillance of Antimicrobial Resistance (network)
CDC	United States Centers for Disease Control and Prevention
CINDI	Countrywide Integrated Noncommunicable Diseases Intervention (network)
CIS	Commonwealth of Independent States

EC	European Commission
ECDC	European Centre for Disease Prevention and Control
EFSA	European Food Safety Authority
EMCA	European Mosquito Control Association
EMCDDA	European Monitoring Centre for Drugs and Drug Addiction
ESCMID	European Society of Clinical Microbiology and Infectious Diseases
EU	European Union
Eurostat	statistical office of the European Union
EVIPNet	Evidence-Informed Policy Network
FAO	Food and Agriculture Organization of the United Nations
GPG	(WHO) Global Policy Group
HPA	Health Protection Agency (United Kingdom)
IAEA	International Atomic Energy Agency
ICMM	International Committee of Military Medicine
ILO	International Labour Organization
IOM	International Organization for Migration
JLN	Joint Learning Network for Universal Health Coverage
KIT	Royal Tropical Institute (Netherlands)
NGO	nongovernmental organization
NIS	newly independent states
OECD	Organisation for Economic Co-operation and Development
OHCHR	Office of the High Commissioner for Human Rights
PBAC	Programme, Budget and Administration Committee (of the WHO Executive Board)
RCC	European Regional Certification Commission for Poliomyelitis Eradication
RCM	(United Nations) Regional Coordination Mechanism
Rio+20	United Nations Conference on Sustainable Development
RIVM	National Institute for Public Health and the Environment (Netherlands)
RVC	European Regional Verification Commission for Measles and Rubella Elimination
SCRC	Standing Committee of the Regional Committee
SEEHN	South-eastern Europe Health Network
UNAIDS	Joint United Nations Programme on HIV/AIDS
UNDG	United Nations Development Group
UNDP	United Nations Development Programme
UNECE	United Nations Economic Commission for Europe
UNFPA	United Nations Population Fund
UNHCR	Office of the United Nations High Commissioner for Refugees
UNICEF	United Nations Children's Fund
UNITAID	a global health initiative

UNODC	United Nations Office on Drugs and Crime
USAID	United States Agency for International Development
VBORNET	European Network for Arthropod Vector Surveillance for Human Public Health

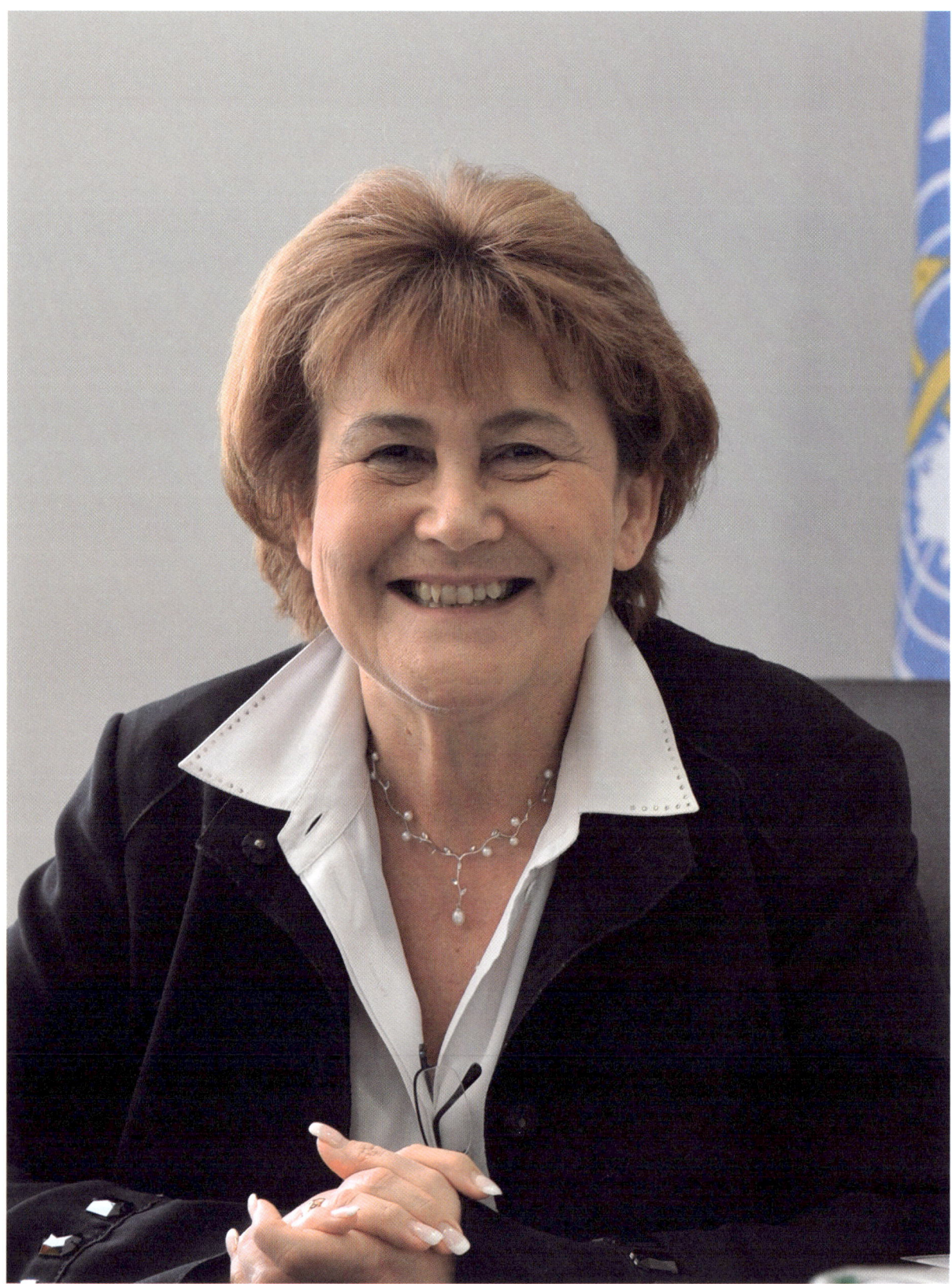

INTRODUCTION: PURSUING BETTER HEALTH FOR EUROPE

Zsuzsanna Jakab

When I took office as WHO Regional Director for Europe in 2010, I proposed an ambitious five-year vision of better health in the WHO European Region (1), and Member States adopted it at the sixtieth session of the WHO Regional Committee for Europe (2). The WHO Regional Office for Europe and the 53 countries it serves therefore agreed to follow a roadmap with specific milestones, to enable the Regional Office to respond to the changing European environment and to further strengthen it as an evidence-based centre of health policy and public health excellence that could better support the Region's diverse Member States (1).

No single publication could tell the whole story of our work and achievements over the last four years. These required great effort, commitment and cooperation from all of us: the Secretariat and Member States that comprise WHO in Europe, which in turn is part of one WHO worldwide, and all WHO's partners in the Region. Several publications (2–5) give highlights of the first two years of our journey together. This book, my second report as Regional Director, covers the second two years, which include the halfway point of the period covered by the vision (1). It describes how we are making our vision a reality to secure better health for everyone in Europe.

Priorities and challenges

Since 2010, working with countries and a wide range of partners, the Regional Office has pursued seven overarching and interrelated priorities to realize its five-year vision *(1–5)*:

1. developing a European health policy as a coherent policy framework that addresses all the challenges to better health in the Region (including the underlying root causes) through both rejuvenated work on public health and continued work on health systems;
2. improving governance in the WHO European Region and in the Regional Office;
3. further strengthening collaboration with Member States;
4. engaging in strategic partnerships for health and creating improved policy coherence;
5. reviewing Regional Office functions, offices and networks;
6. reaching out through improved information and communications; and
7. promoting the Regional Office as an organization with a positive working environment and sustainable funding for its work.

This report shows that work was either completed or well advanced in all these areas in the 2012–2013 biennium *(6,7)*. While different sections of this report address some of the priorities specifically, work on many of them frames or underlies a wide range of the activities of the WHO Regional Office for Europe.

The driving force for all these activities is the health situation in the Region. The 2012 edition of the Regional Office's flagship publication, the European health report, details this situation *(8)*. It describes how, although the Region has gained five years' life expectancy, which is a tremendous success, inequalities in health – between men and women, groups within countries and countries in the Region – not only persist but also are growing. These, along with gaps in health system development, led to a twelve-year gap in life expectancy and a threefold gap in estimated disability-adjusted life-years (DALYs) lost per country population. Europe's ageing population – people aged 65 years or more are predicted to comprise over 25% of the total by 2050 – has high expectations of and makes increasing demands on health services, which are stretched thin, in some cases, by the global financial crisis of recent years. Most deaths in the European Region are caused by cardiovascular diseases (CVD), cancer, and injury and violence. These conditions, together with diabetes, lung diseases, bone and joint disorders, and mental illness account for most of the burden of disease. But avoidable illness and death from communicable diseases remain important problems; concern focuses mainly on tuberculosis (TB), HIV/AIDS and other sexually transmitted infections, though recent poliomyelitis (polio), rubella and measles epidemics in Europe re-emphasize the need to sustain or improve surveillance and immunization for better health protection *(8)*.

This report gives highlights of the work of the WHO Regional Office for Europe in addressing all these challenges in 2012–2013. Details of all the Regional Office's activities are available on its website *(9)*.

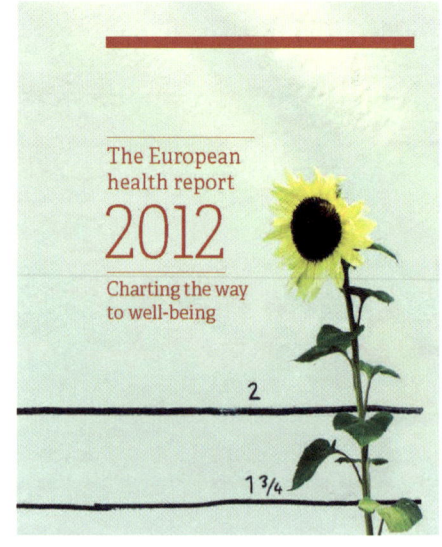

1. TACKLING EUROPE'S HEALTH CHALLENGES AND PRIORITIES

Health 2020: the European policy for health and well-being

In addition to crafting specific responses to the challenges to better health in the Region described in this chapter, the WHO Regional Office for Europe developed the new European health policy, Health 2020, which addresses all of them and links all Regional Office activities. In 2012–2013, the Regional Office completed the development process; the Regional Committee enthusiastically adopted the policy framework, and countries began to implement it with the Regional Office's support *(6,7)*.

Development and adoption
As requested by the Regional Committee *(2,4)*, the Regional Office gathered evidence by consulting hundreds of experts from a wide range of disciplines (through the Internet, at face-to-face events and through such bodies as the Regional Committee, the Standing Committee of the Regional Committee (SCRC) *(10)* and the European Health Policy Forum for High-level Government Officials), documented the experience of policy-makers and public health advocates, and conducted peer reviews among thousands of stakeholders to ensure Health 2020's relevance in different contexts and systems. At the same time, the Regional Office sought evidence to inform the policy and support action for its implementation. It brought the process to fruition by presenting the 2012 Regional Committee with two policy documents, published in one volume in 2013 *(11)*, and a panoply of supporting information on the evidence base, implementation and a monitoring framework *(12–15)*.

The sixty-second session of the Regional Committee eagerly adopted Health 2020 *(6)*. Speakers from 30 countries welcomed its roots in earlier Regional

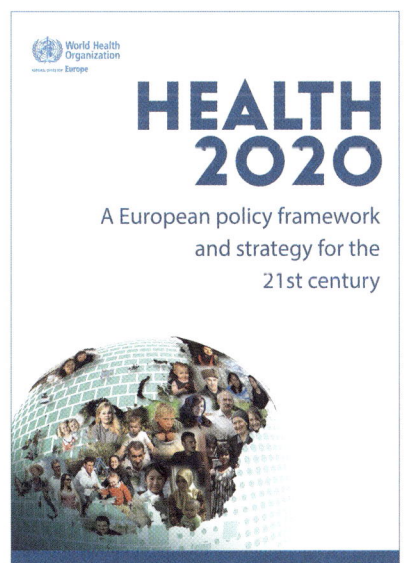

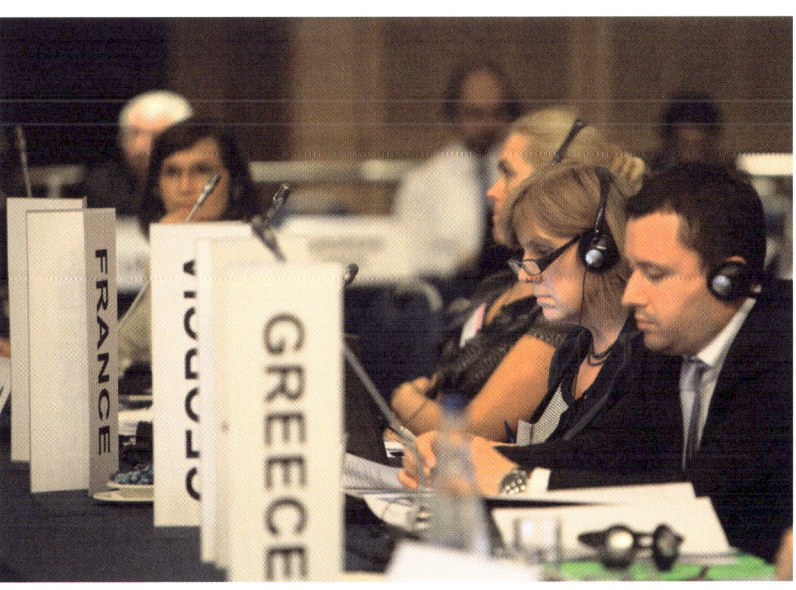

Office policy work (such as policies for health for all and the Tallinn Charter: Health Systems for Health and Wealth *(16)*), alignment with the work for WHO reform, underlying evidence base, advocacy of whole-of-government and -society approaches, and synergy with the new action plan to strengthen public health (see Chapter 2) *(17)* and a range of European Union (EU) policies and programmes. In resolution EUR/RC62/R4 *(18)*, the Regional Committee:

- praised the participatory development process;
- adopted the regional policy framework for health and well-being *(11)* as a guiding framework for health policy development in the Region, including a few regional targets and indicators relevant to all Member States;
- welcomed the European health policy framework and strategy *(11)* as a source of evidence-based guidance on policies and actions to implement Health 2020;
- called on Member States to consider Health 2020 when developing and updating their policies for health development; and
- asked the WHO Regional Director for Europe to develop a monitoring system for Health 2020 for submission to the 2013 Regional Committee.

Health 2020 was crafted as a strategy for action and innovation in national health policies, providing practical solutions to public health challenges that were based on evidence and information, and enabling the comparison of policies and strategies among countries. It promotes processes and mechanisms to engage other sectors in health in all policies, whole-of-government and whole-of-society approaches as means of developing health and resilience and empowering communities. The evidence base legitimized action, thereby providing a basis for political commitment, and made the case for the moral and economic aspects of health. Health 2020 is a valuable tool for a range of actors in health:

- indicating new leadership roles and opportunities for ministers of health;
- identifying ways to make an economic case for investment in health for government leaders;
- outlining integrative strategies and interventions for health professionals to address the major health challenges in the Region, to link these with equity and the social determinants of health and to strengthen health systems;
- basing work with partner agencies on a common set of values, evidence and experience; and
- empowering citizens, consumers and patients for patient-centred care.

Evidence base

Convened by the Regional Office, a group of experts drafted Health 2020 and its support documents, using the best available evidence, systematically reviewed and collated. The process was fully participatory, involving Member States and partners throughout the development phase. To support this work, the Regional Office mapped the best solutions to public health challenges in the European Region and opportunities to promote health and well-being, and commissioned or adopted five studies, published in 2012–2013. These studies provide evidence supporting the effectiveness of Health 2020's objectives, approaches and strategies.

1. Chaired by Professor Sir Michael Marmot, supported by a secretariat at University College London, United Kingdom and drawing on the work of 13 task groups, the review of the social determinants of health and the health divide in the WHO European Region analysed health inequities between and within European countries and recommended policy options for immediate action on health inequities in low-, middle- and high-income countries. With results given in a full report and an executive summary *(19,20)* and urging countries to "do something, do more, do better", the review was warmly welcomed by the Regional Committee *(7)* and officially launched in London, United Kingdom in October 2013.

2. The two studies on governance for health in the 21st century, led by Professor Ilona Kickbusch, reviewed new, collaborative approaches to governance that were driven by the changing nature of current challenges, showed the need for whole-of-government and -society approaches to secure overarching societal goals (such as prosperity, well-being, equity and sustainability) and proposed five types of smart governance for health *(21, 22)*.
3. The study of intersectoral governance for health presented analysis of and experience with the use of structures for intersectoral governance (ranging from committees to financing arrangements and means of engaging the public and industry) to ensure the consideration of Health in All Policies *(23)*.
4. The European Observatory on Health Systems and Policies, a partnership hosted by the Regional Office, and the Organisation for Economic Co-operation and Development (OECD) collated evidence on the economic case for investing in public health actions, including the case for investment before health care services are required, and showed the need for wide-ranging preventive strategies, addressing multiple determinants of health across social groups, as cost-effective means of tackling chronic diseases through interventions to modify lifestyle risk factors *(24)*.
5. Finally, the WHO Regional Office for Europe reviewed and analysed the commitments made between 1990 and 2010 in Regional Committee resolutions, policy statements from conferences and legally binding instruments, such as the International Health Regulations (IHR), the Protocol on Water and Health and the WHO Framework Convention on Tobacco Control. It aimed to support the development of Health 2020 and facilitate its implementation as a reframing of previous commitments within a coherent and visionary approach *(25)*.

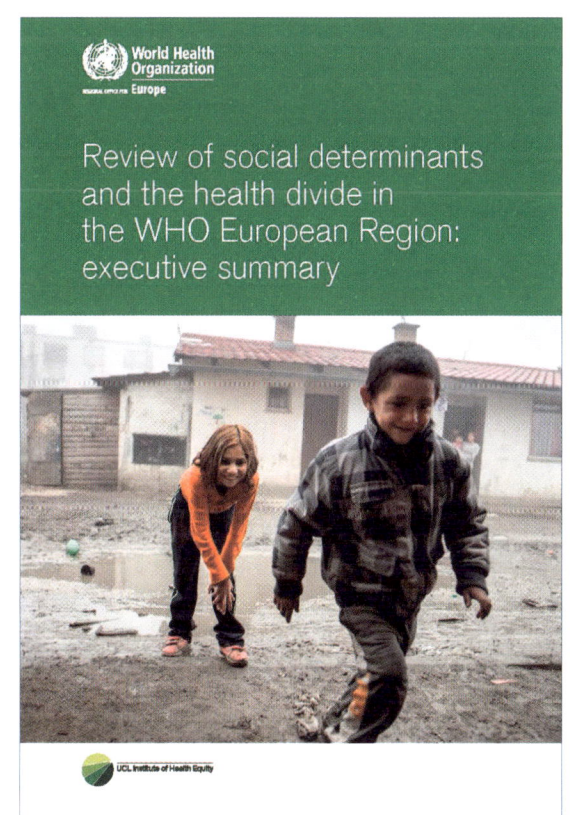

Implementation

The WHO Regional Office for Europe supported the adoption and adaptation of Health 2020 approaches in countries, which began using them in policy-making during the development phase, through means including an interactive website *(26)*. This work focused on three major areas: using high-profile events to launch Health 2020 and raise awareness at the national and international levels, aligning the Regional Office's work to support countries in the current and next biennia, and applying a Health 2020 lens to its programmatic work, as shown below. The Regional Office concentrated on types of support with maximum impact, including intercountry mechanisms and online learning forums to supplement country-based activities.

The Regional Office developed an integrated implementation package to help Member States introduce Health 2020 to sectors other than health, and develop whole-of-government and life-course approaches *(27)*. The core package of resources and

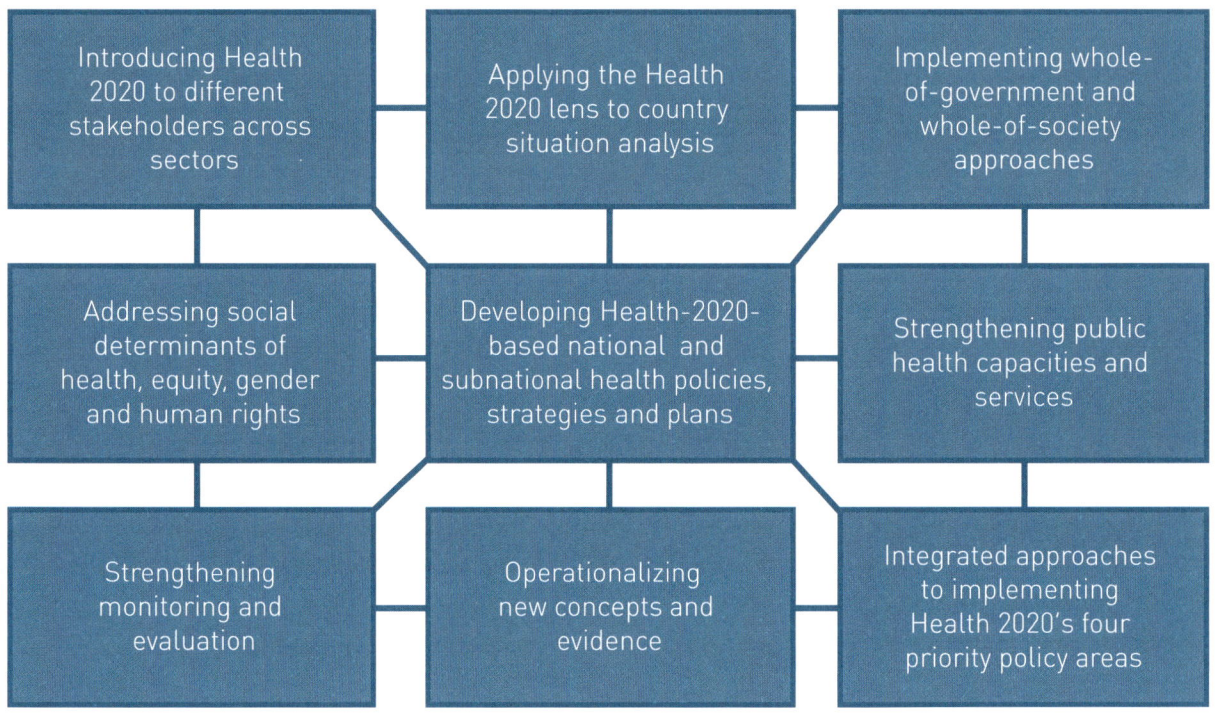

services was intended to promote understanding of both Health 2020 as a whole and its components, to support the development and implementation of national and subnational policy addressing Health 2020's two strategic objectives and four policy priorities, and to support capacity building for implementation, the development of partnerships and the monitoring of progress across the Region. This package has nine components, including: introducing the policy to other sectors, drawing up national health policies, introducing intersectoral and life-course approaches, systematically addressing inequalities and strengthening health systems and public health services.

Countries showed their enthusiasm for Health 2020 by the variety and volume of their implementation activities (7,27). They found it a powerful tool in improving health, reducing health inequalities and strengthening leadership and governance for health. Many countries' health-system priorities mirrored its goals. Stimulated by the policy framework, countries adopted innovative policies, especially for vulnerable groups such as children and people aged over 50. The policy provided useful guidance when the economic crisis necessitated reforms to health care systems. Focusing efforts on health promotion and disease prevention generated well-being and fostered social cohesion, while contributing to the sustainability of health systems in the medium and long terms. Developing community services and extending health insurance coverage were also found to be cost-effective measures. Examples of implementation activities at various levels that were discussed by the 2013 Regional Committee (27) included:

- setting targets (Austria);
- applying a whole-of-government approach to policy-making (Ireland);
- undertaking national consensus-building conferences (Latvia and Lithuania) and making national policies fully aligned with Health 2020 (Switzerland);
- making a Health 2020 growth strategy (countries of the South-eastern Europe Health Network (SEEHN));

- continuing to forge more intersectoral collaboration for health (Turkey); and
- establishing a national centre for disease prevention and control (Ukraine).

To help the Regional Office support countries' implementation work, the SCRC formed a subgroup on Health 2020 in late 2013 *(10)*. It would advise the Regional Office on issues that could arise in implementation and ways to mobilize populations to implement the strategy. At its first meeting, the subgroup identified several priority issues: implementing multisectoral action and national health policies, strengthening public health, promoting training in Health 2020 for multidisciplinary health workers, and streamlining integrated monitoring and reporting on all aspects of Health 2020.

The Regional Office went into 2014 preparing to increase its capacity to meet the high demand from Member States for support and advice, by training a first group of consultants on Health 2020 *(28)*. These would be public health experts from across the WHO European Region who would be expected to work with countries for at least two years.

Targets and indicators: measuring health and well-being

Further to support Health 2020 implementation, the Regional Office developed both targets for the Region and indicators to use in measuring progress towards achieving them, including indicators for the previously unmeasured domain of well-being.

In 2012, the Regional Committee agreed on six overarching targets for Health 2020 *(6)*.

1. Reduce premature mortality in Europe.
2. Increase life expectancy in Europe.
3. Reduce inequities in health in Europe.
4. Enhance the well-being of the European population.
5. Provide universal coverage in Europe.
6. Establish national targets set by Member States.

This was the end of a broad consultative process to secure specific, measurable, achievable, relevant and timely (SMART) targets. Member States provided detailed input, particularly through three meetings of the European Health Policy Forum for High-level Government Officials, concluding in April 2012 in Belgium *(29)*, and a working group established under the SCRC *(10)*. This working

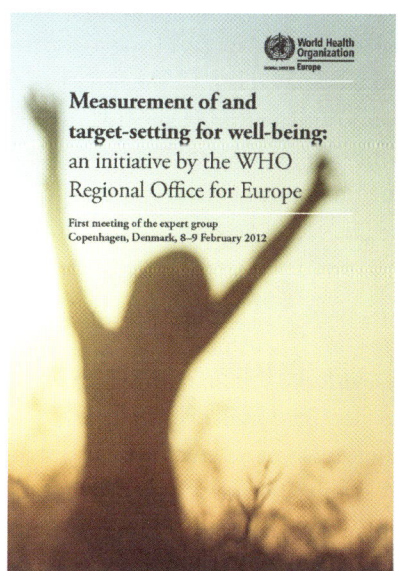
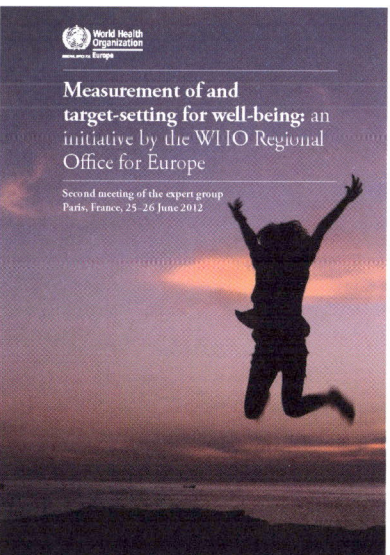
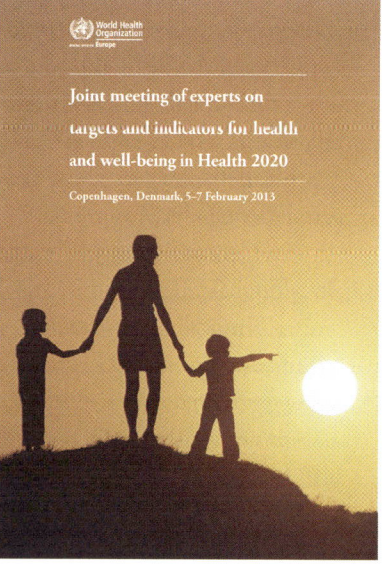

group and extensive written and face-to-face country consultation winnowed the initial list of 51 targets to the 6 approved by the SCRC in May 2012 and the Regional Committee in September.

To provide indicators to measure progress towards the targets, the Regional Office broke new ground in 2012–2013: trying for the first time to map and measure well-being *(8,12,30–32)*. It convened two expert groups, addressing the measurement of well-being and Health 2020 indicators. At a joint meeting in February 2013, these and the SCRC working group on targets for Health 2020 put forward 17 indicators for the 6 targets, including 1 on subjective well-being (life satisfaction) *(32)*. These indicators were based primarily on data routinely provided by countries, and were in line with the global framework for monitoring noncommunicable diseases (NCDs) *(33)*. The Regional Office would report regional averages of the data provided in various information products, including the annual report of the Regional Director, a new annual publication on core health indicators *(34)* and a new, Region-wide health information platform that was planned to be set up in 2014 (through a project with the EU described below).

The Regional Office started consultation on the indicators with Member States in April 2013, and submitted the full list to the sixty-third session of the Regional Committee. Country representatives welcomed the steps taken to harmonize data requirements, rely on existing data and avoid double reporting, as well as the creation of a unified European information system *(7)*, and the Regional Committee adopted the indicators and asked the Regional Office to complete that on objective well-being, implement the proposed monitoring framework *(27)* and regularly collect, analyse and publish information on countries' progress *(35)*. Work on indicators of objective well-being was expected to be completed by April 2014.

Other work for equity and health development

Vulnerable social groups

In addition to making equity the core of Health 2020, the WHO Regional Office for Europe worked to reduce health inequities affecting vulnerable social groups. For example, its new programme on vulnerability and health worked to realize the right to health of women and marginalized populations, and the Regional Office designated a WHO Collaborating Centre on Vulnerability and Health at the University of Debrecen, Hungary, in February 2012 *(36)*.

In 2012–2013, the WHO European Region, particularly the countries closest to North Africa and the Middle East, continued to face large influxes of migrants, which can pose significant health challenges to both migrants and receiving countries. In response, the Regional Office established the Public Health Aspects of Migration in Europe (PHAME) project *(37)*. Supported by Belgium and Italy, the PHAME project worked within the Health 2020 framework to help countries make systematic and evidence-based responses to the public health needs of migrants. This included:

- identifying best practices and engaging in a cross-national political dialogue on migration;
- identifying and filling potential gaps in the delivery of health service, including those for the prevention, diagnosis, monitoring and management of disease;
- supporting the work of policy-makers, health planners, and local health professionals and others responsible for providing high-quality health care to migrants; and
- strengthening countries' national and local capacities to deal with the public health aspects of migration.

In 2012–2013, a WHO team conducted assessment missions in three Member States, in cooperation with their health ministries, that had received or might receive large undocumented populations: Italy, Malta and Portugal. The aim was to coordinate the health response by identifying best practices and potential gaps in the public health sector before establishing contingency plans.

In addition, the Regional Office helped to strengthen the health components of national strategies for Roma integration and policy and action plans for the EU Decade of Roma Inclusion 2005–2015 by such means as supporting the Roma Health Fund, a nongovernmental organization (NGO) *(38)* and publishing a quarterly newsletter in cooperation with the European Commission (EC) Directorate-General for Health and Consumers and the University of Alicante, Spain *(39)*. In late 2013, the Regional Office published a case study that gave a critical overview of the Roma health mediation programme in Romania *(40)*. The case study was produced to inform a resource package for health professionals to be used in multicountry capacity-building events; like many activities focusing on Roma health, it was carried out within the framework of work towards the Millennium Development Goals (MDGs).

MDGs and the post-2015 development agenda

The Regional Office supported countries' efforts to achieve the health-related MDGs through its technical programmes, reported on progress towards achieving MDGs 4–6 *(41)* and, with the WHO Collaborating Centre on Social Inclusion and Health at the University of Alicante and the Spanish Ministry of Health, Social Services and Equality, organized a training course on reorienting work to achieve MDGs 4 and 5 for greater health equity for Roma people for public health experts from Albania, Bosnia and Herzegovina, Bulgaria, Montenegro, Serbia and the former Yugoslav Republic of Macedonia. The Regional Office led two United Nations interagency working groups coordinating action towards MDG achievement: on the health of Roma women and children and on tackling inequities. This was part of an interagency coordination initiative involving

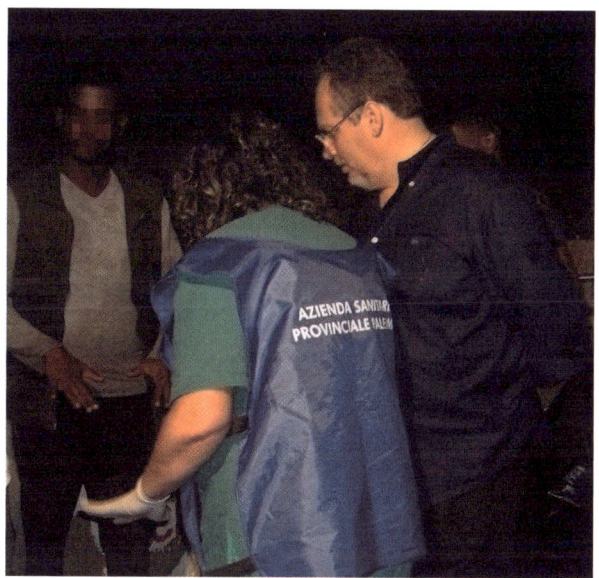

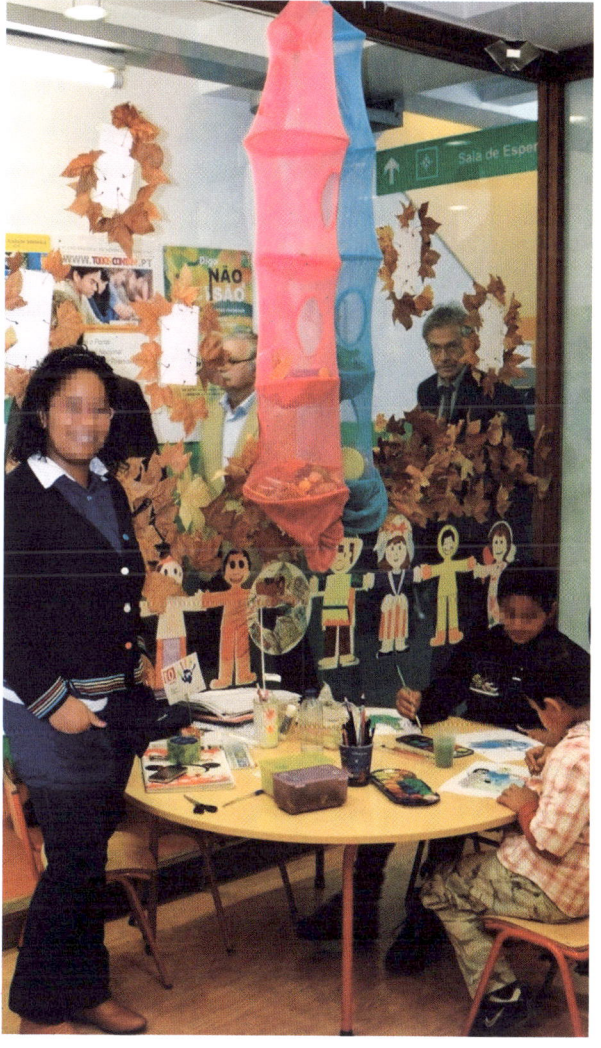

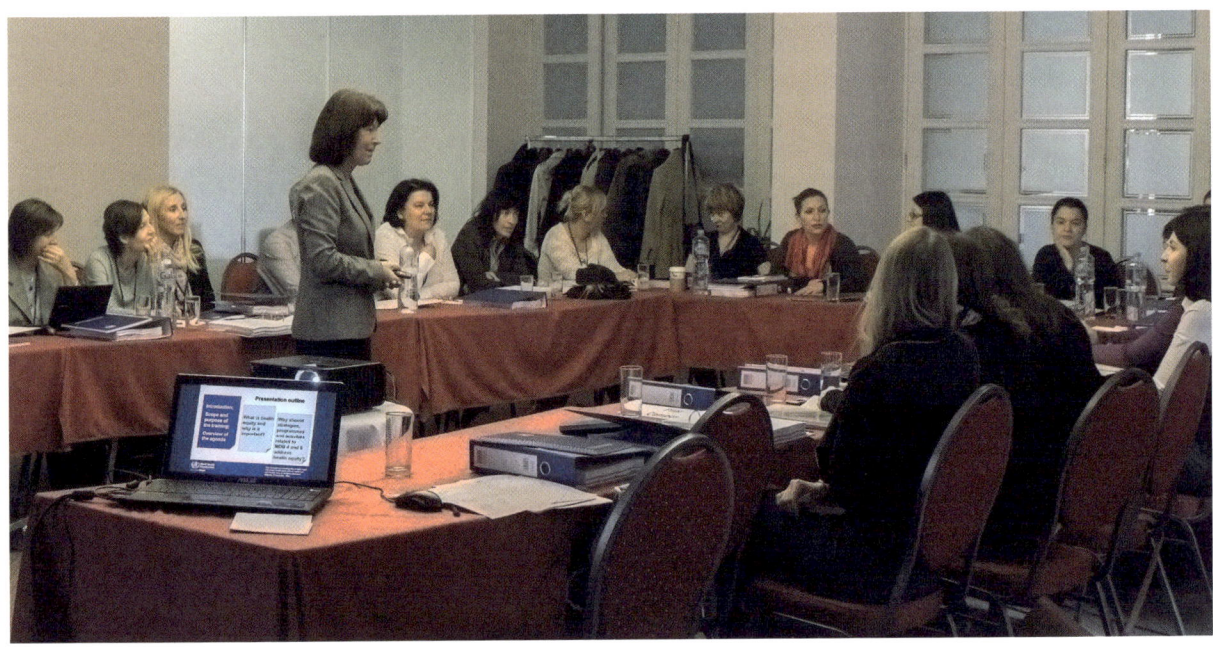

the United Nations Population Fund (UNFPA), the Office of the High Commissioner for Human Rights (OHCHR), the United Nations Development Programme (UNDP), the United Nations Children's Fund (UNICEF) and the International Organization for Migration (IOM) (42).

Further, the WHO Regional Director for Europe signed a framework for action with the UNFPA Regional Director for Eastern Europe and Central Asia and the UNICEF Regional Director for Central and Eastern Europe and the Commonwealth of Independent States at the 2013 session of the Regional Committee (7). Their joint aim was to more effectively support Member States in achieving MDGs 4–6, and address new challenges in the Region in the context of Health 2020. In the framework for action, the three agencies committed themselves to consolidating their work to improve the quality of health care delivery for women and children and to ensure universal health coverage, especially for underserved and vulnerable populations. The framework also contained priorities for bilateral action and made a commitment to strengthen mutual accountability and monitoring of implementation.

Finally, the Regional Office was closely engaged in the process of determining the development agenda after 2015 (the deadline for achieving the MDGs) to ensure that health is positioned as a critical contributor to and outcome of sustainable development and human well-being (6,7). Its strategy was to support Member States in their participation in the negotiations at the United Nations. In addition, the Regional Director took part in discussions of this topic at meetings of United Nations regional directors in Switzerland in October 2012 and Denmark in March 2013. A regional United Nations interagency advocacy package was prepared, describing the main achievements and challenges faced in Europe with the MDGs and setting a vision for health after 2015. Albania, Armenia, Azerbaijan, Kazakhstan, Montenegro, the Republic of Moldova, Serbia, Tajikistan, Turkey and Ukraine, plus Kosovo (in accordance with Security Council resolution 1244 (1999)), conducted consultations on the post-2015 development agenda.

To help formulate the message that the WHO governing bodies would contribute to the United Nations deliberations on the post-2015 agenda, the 2013 Regional Committee agreed that health should be a priority, with a focus on maximizing health for all throughout the life-course and universal health coverage as both a means to that end and an end in itself (7). Universal health coverage was essential to the integrated approach and government- and society-wide action, including on social determinants, required to improve health.

In November 2013, the Regional Office helped to organize a multistakeholder regional consultation in Istanbul, Turkey on the post-2015 development agenda, in partnership with the United Nations Development Group (UNDG) Europe and Central Asia and the Regional Coordination Mechanism (RCM), led by UNDP and the United Nations Economic Commission for Europe (UNECE), and hosted by the Ministry of Development of Turkey. The participants – representing governments, international organizations, civil society, the private sector, academe and the mass media – stressed the critical role of health in the post-2015 agenda, both as an outcome of and determinant of sustainable development and poverty eradication, and called Health 2020 (11) crucial for setting the ground and formulating a new vision for health in this context.

2. STRENGTHENING HEALTH SYSTEMS

Europe's health challenges and the pressures exerted by the financial crisis highlighted the need for comprehensive responses from health systems, working towards universal coverage with evidence-informed policies. Strengthening people-centred health systems is one of the four pillars of Health 2020 *(11)*.

Action plan to rejuvenate public health

Emphasizing public health as an essential component of health systems, the WHO Regional Office for Europe developed the European Action Plan for Strengthening Public Health Capacities and Services *(17)*, to strengthen public health functions, infrastructure and capacity for health protection, disease prevention and health promotion in an integrated approach, including primary health care. The Action Plan encompassed 10 essential public health operations, grouped for the integrated delivery of services, and provided a self-assessment tool that each country could use to identify any gaps in areas of work or funding. The Plan will be implemented between 2012 and 2020, with continued consultation with Member States, experts and working groups; a governance structure; and a steering group.

The Action Plan is at the heart of Health 2020 and its implementation; like the new policy, it is in line with WHO reform, will support implementation of the Tallinn Charter *(16)* and was developed through a process of wide consultation with, for example, civil-society and health professionals' organizations, and through numerous meetings at the subregional, regional and global levels. In addition, the Regional Office based the Plan on solid evidence, including assessments of public health services and capacity in 41 of the 53 countries in the WHO European Region, a study on institutional models and funding structures for delivering essential public health operations, and a study on tools and instruments for legislation and policy on public health *(43–45)*. The 2012 Regional Committee strongly endorsed the Action Plan, calling on countries and international partners to implement it, and asking the Regional Director to further develop its essential public health operations and self-assessment tool, and to report back on this and the implementation of the Action Plan in 2016 *(6)*.

As with Health 2020, countries began using the tools and implementing the Plan during the development process, and the Regional Office supported countries' implementation efforts after its adoption. This included promoting the Action Plan at meetings of SEEHN in December 2012 and the International Network of Health Promoting Hospitals and Health Services in January 2013, and helping countries such as Estonia, Greece, the Republic of Moldova, the former Yugoslav Republic of Macedonia and Ukraine to use it in developing new national public health strategies and legislation (45,46).

Comprehensive responses from health systems

Universal health coverage was the key policy direction in the Regional Office's work to strengthen people-centred health systems (46). Many countries had achieved substantial progress in providing their populations with financial protection and access to high-quality health services, but 19 million people in the Region were still subject to out-of-pocket health expenditure that placed a catastrophic burden on their households.

In 2012–2013, the Regional Office supported countries with a range of products and services to promote policies that help them move towards or sustain universal coverage. It offered tailored advisory services and policy dialogues in Member States on key issues in health financing policy, developed lessons and policy recommendations to strengthen health systems' resilience, and conducted national, regional and multicountry training to build countries' capacities (47). It also worked to strengthen health systems' workforces, and revived its programme on nursing and midwifery.

To strengthen the second pillar of universal health coverage, the Regional Office started development of the Framework for Action towards Coordinated/Integrated Health Services Delivery, which would support countries with policy options and recommendations to strengthen the coordination/integration of health services. It began by making a roadmap setting out the phases up to 2016 and giving particular attention to ensuring the participation of partners, including focal points in countries, external experts and leading organizations such as the International Foundation for Integrated Care (48). The Regional Office launched this workplan for the Framework at a high-level meeting in October 2013 in Estonia, marking the fifth anniversary of the signing of the Tallinn Charter (16), which called for greater investment in health systems.

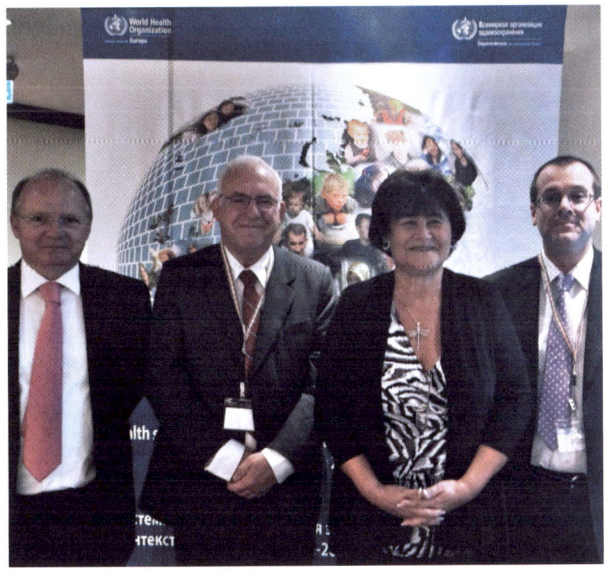
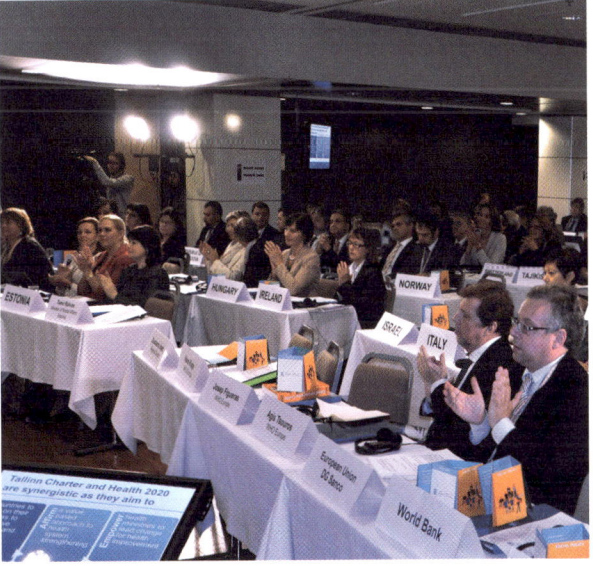

At the meeting in Tallinn, ministers, experts and representatives from 38 Member States, and representatives of key partners (including the EC, OECD, the World Bank and the Global Fund to Fight AIDS, Tuberculosis and Malaria) explained the steps they had taken to implement the Tallinn Charter, and to move towards providing universal health coverage. In addition, ministries had focused more on improving accountability and governance through, for example, assessing the performance of their health systems *(49)*. They identified multiple challenges in this work, and acknowledged key areas for attention in strengthening health systems to provide more people-centred care:

- strengthening the public's health literacy;
- improving the coordination of service provision across all levels;
- focusing on primary care and community care as the cornerstones for the holistic delivery of services with clear links to public health services; and
- investing in health-system inputs, including information sharing and the skill set and competences of staff, to complement more coordinated delivery models for health services.

In addition, the Regional Office also worked to support countries' health systems in improving their use of pharmaceuticals and health technology. Efforts focused on developing and monitoring comprehensive national policies on access to and the quality and rational use of essential medical products and technologies. The Regional Office shared evidence on, promoted and provided training in the use of best practices for increasing and sustaining access to essential, quality medical products. Cooperation with national authorities and other stakeholders took the forms of, for example, a network for the prudent use of antibiotics; assessments in Hungary, Kyrgyzstan, the Republic of Moldova and Tajikistan on access to medicines for treatment of NCDs; stronger cooperation between countries to strengthen their capacities for regulation of medical products; and continued support to the networks for pharmaceutical pricing and reimbursement policy and for rational prescribing.

The WHO Regional Director for Europe addressed the international conference to mark the thirty-fifth anniversary of the Declaration of Alma-Ata *(50)* on primary health care, which took place in Almaty, Kazakhstan in November 2013. Attended by high-level representatives of the Government of Kazakhstan, national representatives from 58 countries across the six WHO regions, and international partners, the conference provided an international platform to exchange policy, practice and research in primary health care. The experiences gained since the adoption of the Declaration helped identify the priority challenges to, options for, and lessons learnt in developing primary health care.

Finally, the 2013 Regional Committee agreed to expand the Regional Office's capacity to support Member States by accepting the Government of Kazakhstan's offer to host a new geographically dispersed office (GDO) for primary health care *(7)*.

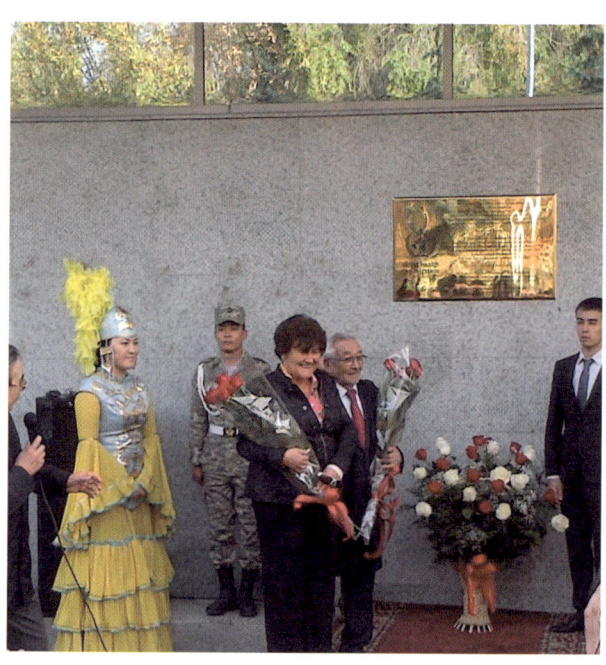

Supporting health system reforms in countries

The Regional Office provided increasing levels of support to Greece *(51)*, starting with technical assistance with national health insurance and the pricing and reimbursement of pharmaceuticals and other public health areas. In July 2013, the Regional Office signed an agreement with the Ministry of Health of Greece to implement the health reform support programme for 2013–2015 in the framework of the Ministry's health in action initiative, which is supported by WHO, the EC Task Force for Greece and the Federal Ministry of Health of Germany. The project is intended to produce a sustainable and equitable health system, ensuring access to high-quality care and financial protection. To guide the reform, Greece would develop a national health strategy outlining a vision for the Greek health system in line with Health 2020. Particularly good progress was made by October on a study on vulnerable populations' access to care and a tool to monitor the effects of the financial crisis on health and the health system in Greece. The Ministry and the Regional Office concluded 2013 by holding a conference on how to boost the country's health sector as part of the health reform, with participants representing the key stakeholders from the Greek and international communities.

The EC Support Group for Cyprus subsequently approached the Regional Office to provide similar assistance as in Greece to their health system reform.

Other examples of the Regional Office's work with countries included support to the Republic of Moldova that took many forms:

- a workshop on the implementation of public–private partnerships in the health sector, with support from the World Bank;
- a flagship course on health system strengthening and sustainable financing;
- a policy dialogue on moving towards universal health coverage by strengthening health financing policies; and
- a review of health financing reforms in the country *(52)*.

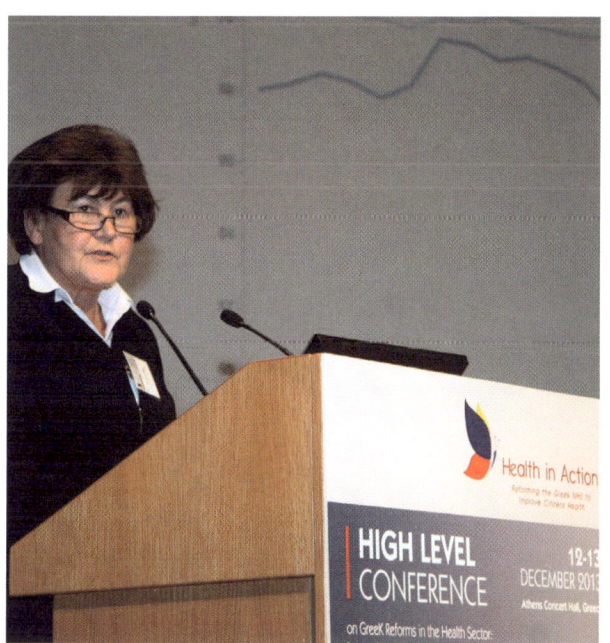
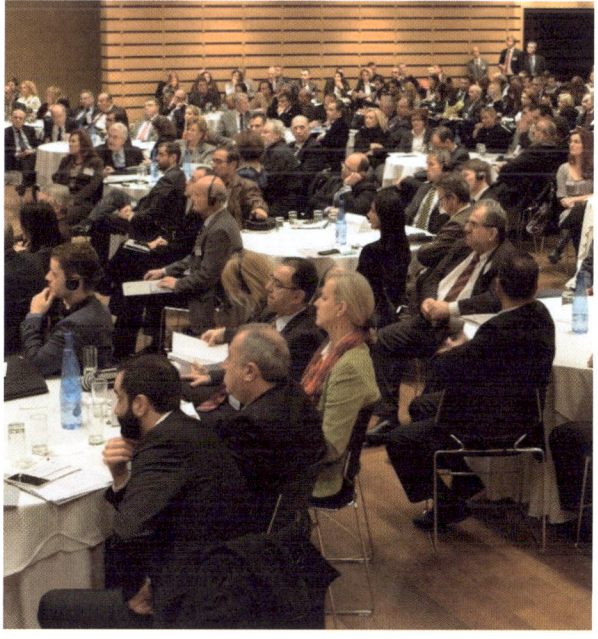

Research on out-of-pocket payments bore fruit in the second half of 2012. The Regional Office published an analysis of the data behind the estimates of such payments in the former USSR in July *(53)* and presented the Armenian Government with the findings of a two-year research project on out-of-pocket health payments, which were used in discussions to further improve financial protection for Armenian citizens, in December. As part of a series of activities supported by WHO headquarters and the United Kingdom Department for International Development, the Regional Office held a policy seminar in Kyrgyzstan that connected universal coverage with the modernization of service delivery. At the end of the year, it joined with the World Bank and the United States Agency for International Development (USAID) to advise the Government of Georgia on measures to establish a universal benefit package of health services for the population.

Working for the financial sustainability and resilience of health systems

Since the onset of the global economic crisis, the WHO Regional Office for Europe has intensified its engagement with Member States on the financial sustainability of the health systems in three ways:

1. doing analytical work to build the evidence base;
2. fostering policy dialogue and events to disseminate current evidence and share ideas on and experience with policy responses and lessons for the future; and
3. providing technical assistance directly to countries (as discussed above).

The Regional Office launched a new section of its website, outlining its efforts and those of Member States to mitigate the negative impact of the crisis on health and health systems, and containing major publications and guidance materials *(54)*. With the World Bank and the Joint Learning Network for Universal Health Coverage (JLN), the Regional Office started work to develop a diagnostic and assessment guide to support countries making reforms to mechanisms for paying health-service providers in 2012. In addition, the Regional Office and the European Observatory on Health Systems and Policies reported on the Irish health system's responses to financial pressures *(55)*, and drafted a summary of policy responses by European countries *(56)*.

The Regional Office and partners held a range of events to support the exchange of information and ideas on health financing *(54)*. With OECD, it organized a joint meeting on the financial sustainability of health systems in central, eastern and south-eastern Europe, in Tallinn, Estonia in June 2012. This helped strengthen collaboration between health and finance officials, and the Regional Office continued to explore further collaboration with OECD and the EU in this field. Co-hosted by Andorra and with sponsorship from the World Bank and the Catalan health authorities in Spain, the Regional Office coordinated a high-level seminar on the governance of health financing for delegations from

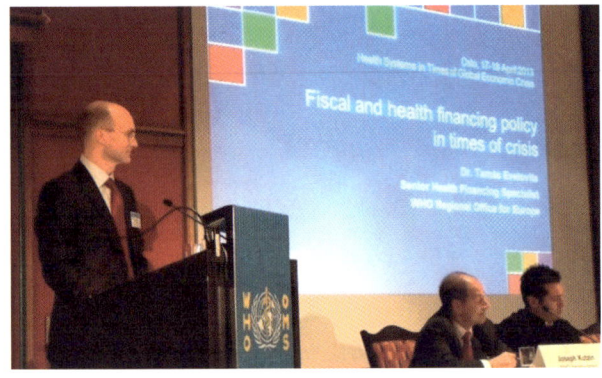
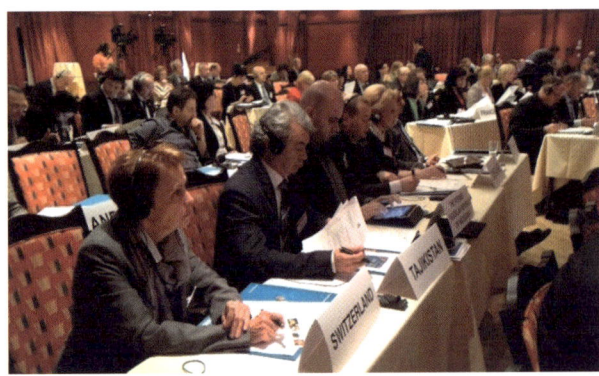

Strengthening health systems

Andorra and Montenegro, in November 2012. It held the ninth Baltic policy dialogue in Latvia in December, focusing on hospital financing and governance, for senior representatives of the health ministries of Estonia, Latvia and Lithuania.

Health ministers discussed policy responses to the economic crisis at the 2012 Regional Committee; work in this area culminated in the conference on health systems in times of global economic crisis, held in April 2013 in Oslo, Norway (57). Four years after Norway hosted the first such event, the Regional Office brought together senior policy-makers from ministries of health and finance; representatives of health insurance funds, patients' organizations and international partners; and researchers, to examine the situation across the Region. The participants reviewed the effects of the crisis on health systems, took stock of government policy responses and assessed the overall impact on health-system outcomes. They considered the summary of policy responses by European Member States (56) and an in-depth examination of selected countries, and reached broad agreement on 10 policy lessons and recommendations needed to address the health impact of the economic crisis. Participants called for a focus on areas and services that encourage economic growth and reinforce solidarity and equity (58). Consultations with Member States and the SCRC further refined the 10 policy lessons and recommendations (59), which were endorsed by the 2013 Regional Committee (7).

Training to build capacity

The Regional Office's major training activities included the second and third sessions of the Barcelona Course on Health Financing, held in May 2012 and 2013 (60). This was an advanced course for professionals seeking to deepen their understanding of options for health financing policy, and it was built around five modules: designing a benefit package, raising revenues, pooling health revenues, purchasing and coordinating reform efforts. Its special theme was moving towards and sustaining universal coverage, highlighting how to counter the impact of economic downturns.

With the World Bank Institute and the Health Policy Analysis Centre of Kyrgyzstan, the Regional Office offered the Flagship Course on Health System Strengthening, focusing on NCDs, in September and October 2012, attended by 50 senior officials and health-sector stakeholders from Albania, Armenia, Azerbaijan, Bulgaria, Kazakhstan, the Republic of Moldova, Romania, the Russian Federation, Serbia, Spain, Tajikistan, Turkey, Ukraine and Uzbekistan. In addition, OECD, WHO headquarters and the WHO Regional Office for Europe held a technical workshop on the implementation of the health financing framework under the System of Health Accounts for OECD, EU and EU accession countries in Paris, France in October 2012. The tenth Flagship Course, addressing the same topics, was held in October 2013; it had modules on the health policy cycle and

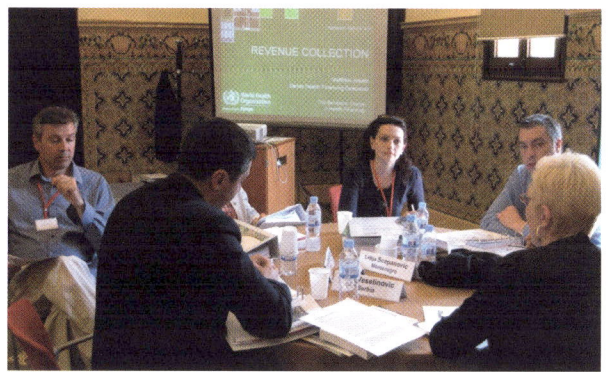
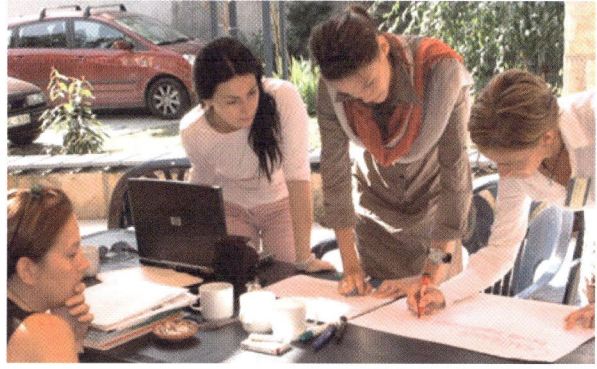

health system performance, the organization of health services for populations and individuals, and health financing *(61)*.

Seeking a skilled and sustainable health workforce

The Regional Office focused on capacity building in and the sustainability of the health workforce *(62)*. This work included a three-day capacity-building workshop for paediatricians in April 2012 in Tajikistan, and a technical meeting to strengthen the health workforce knowledge base to support evidence-informed health policies in June in the Republic of Moldova. The latter was organized by the WHO Regional Office for Europe in collaboration with SEEHN and hosted by the Ministry of Health of the Republic of Moldova, and drew participants from Albania, Bosnia and Herzegovina, Bulgaria, Croatia, Israel, Montenegro, the Republic of Moldova, Romania, Serbia and the former Yugoslav Republic of Macedonia. In June 2013, the Regional Office, with the Ministry of Health and the National Health Insurance Company of the Republic of Moldova, held a policy dialogue on performance-related payment at which experts shared the experience of Estonia, Spain and the United Kingdom in this area. The policy dialogue and continuing work to strengthen the Republic of Moldova's health workforce and capacity to manage the migration of Moldovan health professionals were related to an EU-funded project.

With the European Observatory on Health Systems and Policies, the Regional Office held a policy dialogue, in Belarus in August 2012, on new skills and roles for health professionals in countries in the Commonwealth of Independent States (CIS). At the 2012 session of the Regional Committee, it held a technical discussion for representatives from health ministries, international organizations and NGOs on action needed to achieve a sustainable health workforce and strengthen health systems in Europe *(6)*. The WHO regional offices for Europe and the Western Pacific, in cooperation with a WHO collaborating centre and the Royal Tropical Institute (KIT) in Amsterdam, held an international policy dialogue in the Netherlands in May 2013 on challenges to health-workforce mobility and recruitment; the participants agreed on five key messages for the stakeholders in this issue *(63)*.

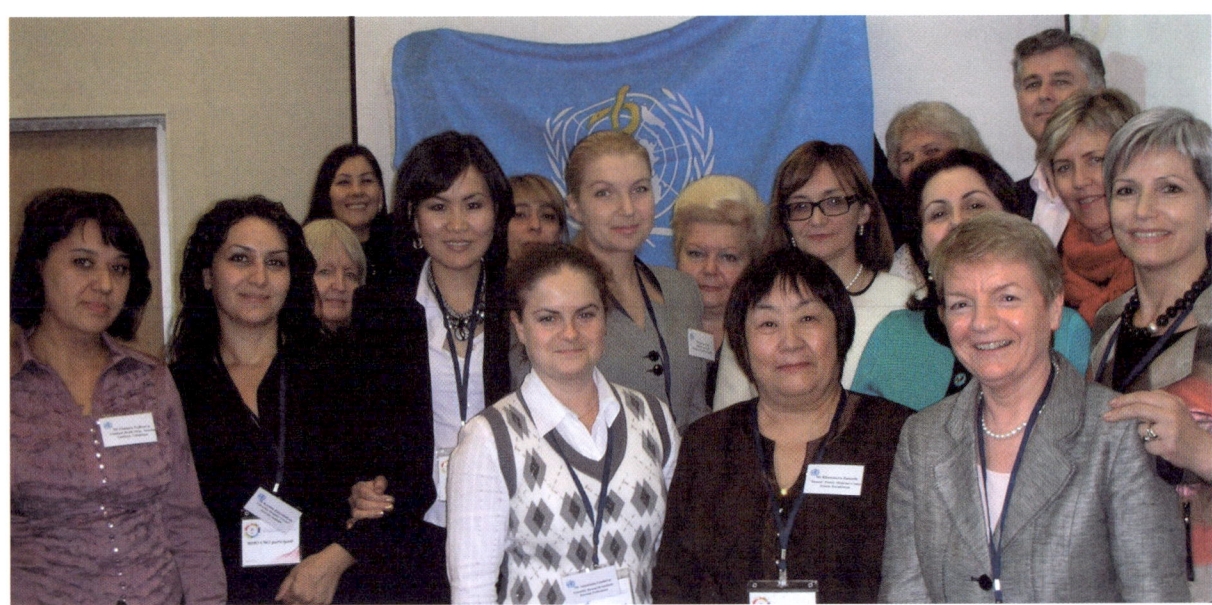

The Regional Office convened meetings of health professionals, including a subregional meeting of chief nursing officers from CIS countries in St Petersburg, the Russian Federation in October 2012 *(62)*. It supported a joint meeting of chief medical, nursing and dental officers held by Cyprus in October 2012, in the context of its EU Presidency. Under Lithuania's EU Presidency, the Regional Office held its second meeting of government chief nursing officers in Vilnius in October 2013. Over 80 participants from 41 countries, including representatives of national nursing and midwifery associations and WHO collaborating centres, met to explore ways to strengthen nursing and midwifery to enhance their contributions to achieving the goals of Health 2020.

Finally, the Regional Office started two major new initiatives on workforce development: to strengthen the public health workforce (in close collaboration with the Association of Schools of Public Health in the European Region (ASPHER) and partners) and to transform the education and training of the health workforce through cooperation between the health, science and education sectors.

Evidence and information for policy-making

As this report shows, providing evidence and information for policy-making forms a major part of nearly all Regional Office activities. Chapter 1 describes work to build the evidence base to support Health 2020, define its goals and construct indicators to measure progress towards achieving them. This section deals with other examples.

Following the roadmap agreed in 2010, the WHO Regional Office for Europe and the EC made good progress in 2012–2013 towards their agreed goal of building a common public health information system for the European Region *(64)*, an initiative endorsed by the 2013 Regional Committee *(7)*. The partners completed the first four steps in 2012–2013:

- mapping their existing health information systems, including databases *(65)*;
- reviewing the quality and architecture of these systems, including devising quality criteria;

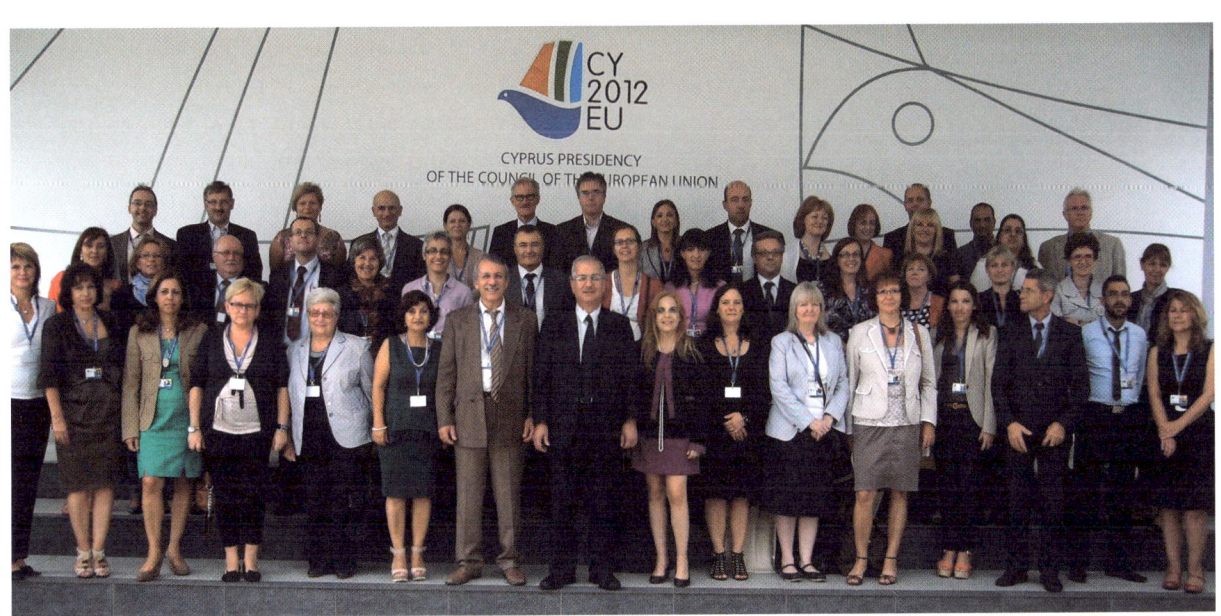

- seeking and bringing on board other potential partners and stakeholders, such as OECD, Eurostat (the statistical office of the EU) and the National Institute for Public Health and the Environment (RIVM) of the Netherlands; and
- defining common needs and constraints.

One step remained for completion in 2014: determining a concrete way forward and devising an action plan.

The partners aimed to further strengthen collaboration by involving the EC Directorate-General for Health and Consumers in the drafting of WHO's European health information strategy and its working group on measuring well-being *(30–32)*, and involving the Regional Office in relevant health information activities led by the Directorate-General.

In addition, the Regional Office maintained and updated its widely used statistical databases and interactive atlases of health inequalities in 2012–2013 *(65)*. It also offered a new resource, the European database on human and technical resources for health *(66)*, in September 2013; the database contains nearly 200 indicators on non-monetary health care resources in all 53 Member States of the WHO European Region. The data were collected jointly by Eurostat, OECD and the Regional Office. Not only does the database provide valuable

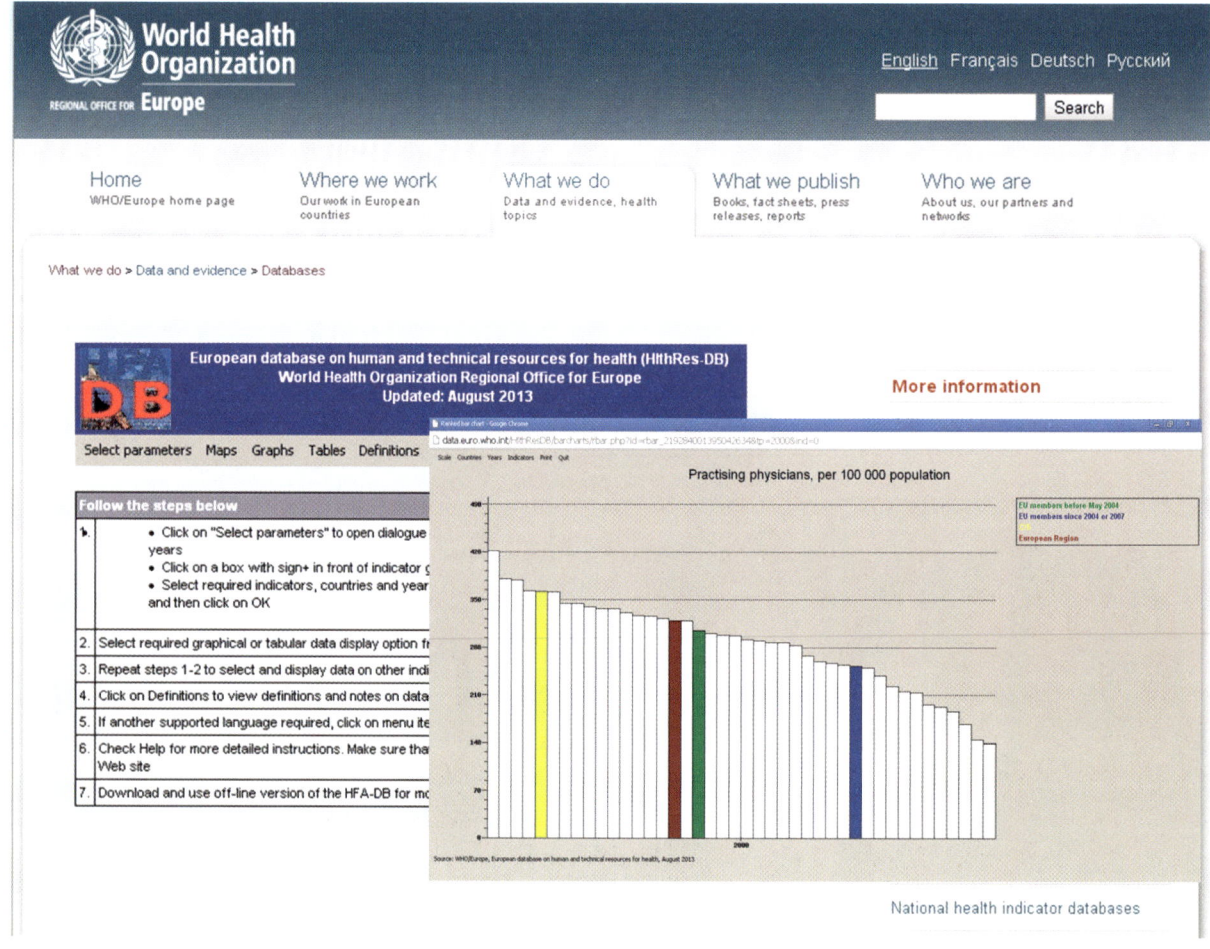

National health indicator databases

Strengthening health systems

information to countries but the joint data collection reduced the reporting burden on them and ensured that the definitions used and information provided were harmonized between the partner organizations.

To further promote the systematic use of health-research evidence in policy-making, the Regional Office launched EVIPNet (the WHO Evidence-Informed Policy Network) in the European Region at a workshop in Bishkek, Kyrgyzstan in October 2012, attended by representatives of Azerbaijan, Kyrgyzstan, Tajikistan and Turkmenistan, along with partner organizations, including the Overseas Development Institute, the United Kingdom, UNFPA and USAID (67).

EVIPNet would organize a series of workshops on the different ways to support evidence-informed health policy across the Region. The Regional Office held the first EVIPNet workshop on evidence-informed policy-making in October 2013 for participants from 15 Member States: Albania, Estonia, Hungary, Kazakhstan, Kyrgyzstan, Lithuania, Poland, the Republic of Moldova, Romania, Slovenia, Tajikistan, the former Yugoslav Republic of Macedonia, Turkey, Turkmenistan and Ukraine. The EVIPNet meeting organized sessions jointly and in parallel with the Autumn School on Health Information and Evidence for Policy-making, held in Izmir, Turkey, a joint venture between the WHO Regional Office for Europe and RIVM (68).

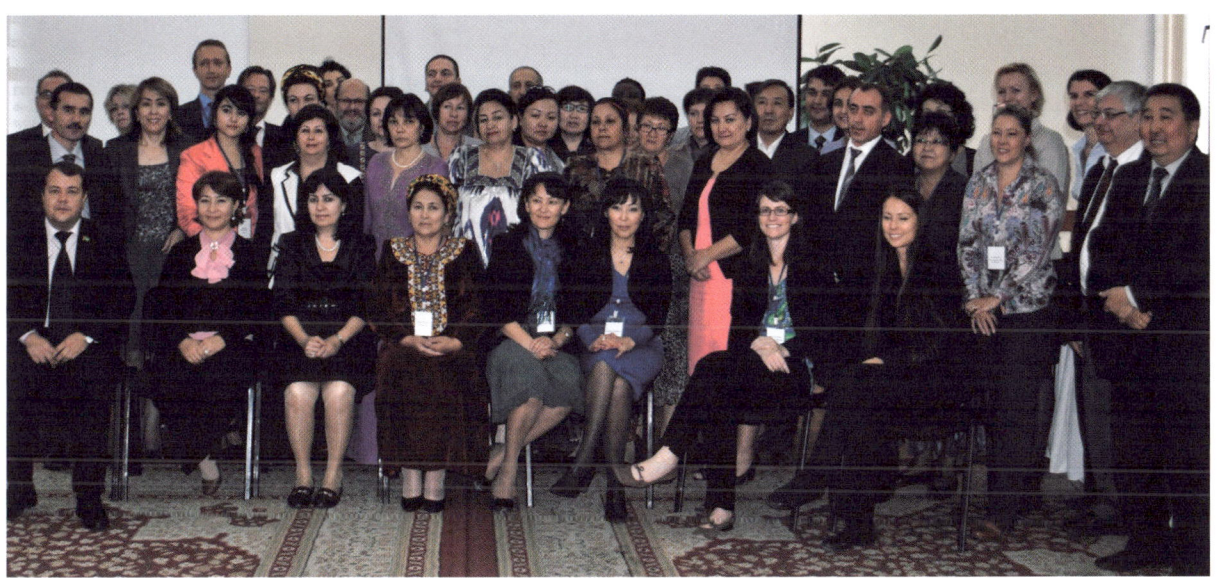

3. NCDs AND PROMOTING HEALTH THROUGHOUT LIFE

In 2012–2013, the WHO Regional Office for Europe pursued the global target on NCDs, adopted by the 2013 World Health Assembly, by both promoting a comprehensive, integrated approach and supporting action on individual risk factors, and worked to promote health throughout the life-course. Its work – particularly on such issues as tobacco, nutrition and physical activity, and mental health – sought to prompt Region-wide responses linked to Health 2020.

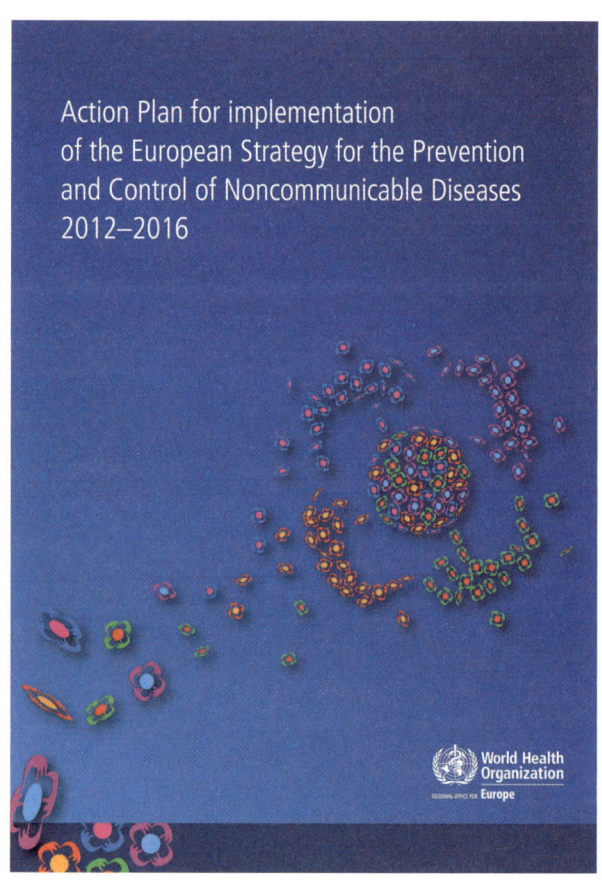

To increase the Regional Office's capacity to assist Member States in their struggle against NCDs, the planned GDO on this topic would be opened in Moscow, the Russian Federation in 2014 *(7)*.

Supporting comprehensive action

The Regional Office started implementing two commitments made in 2011: the Action Plan for implementation of the European Strategy for the Prevention and Control of Noncommunicable Diseases 2012–2016, and the Political Declaration of the United Nations General Assembly *(69,70)*.

As requested by the United Nations high-level meeting on NCD prevention and control, the 2012 World Health Assembly set a global target of a 25% reduction in premature death from NCDs by 2025. The Regional Office conducted a web-based consultation to maximize European Member States' input to the global process of choosing specific targets and indicators for a global monitoring framework for NCDs *(71)*, and the Norwegian Government hosted a consultation on the framework, as well as one on the global and European action plans on mental health. The 2013 World Health Assembly adopted the global framework, comprising 9 global targets and 25 indicators *(33)*.

Work at both the global and regional levels focused on leading NCDs (CVD, cancer, diabetes and chronic respiratory diseases) and their shared risk factors (tobacco use, harmful use of alcohol, physical inactivity and unhealthy diet); the European Action

Plan provides a comprehensive and integrated framework for interventions in four priority action areas *(69)*:

- governance, including building alliances and networks, and fostering citizen empowerment;
- strengthening surveillance, monitoring and evaluation, and research;
- promoting health and preventing disease; and
- reorienting health services further towards prevention and care of chronic diseases.

The Regional Office worked closely with countries and partner organizations to support the Action Plan's implementation. Several European countries strengthened their health information systems by improving the data collected on NCDs. Azerbaijan, Turkey and Uzbekistan implemented the WHO STEPwise approach to surveillance, a simple, standardized method for collecting, analysing and disseminating data on the main risk factors. The Regional Office supported Azerbaijan, Bulgaria, Estonia, Lithuania, the Republic of Moldova and Ukraine in developing strategies and plans on NCDs. Through a project supported by the Government of the Russian Federation, WHO worked intensively with Armenia, Kyrgyzstan, Tajikistan and Uzbekistan to develop NCD strategies and policies, and strengthen their integrated surveillance systems. Through the Programme of Action for Cancer Therapy (PACT), WHO and the International Atomic Energy Agency (IAEA) help countries optimize their investments in cancer prevention and control by assessing and making recommendations on their cancer programmes. In 2012–2013, missions were organized to Armenia, the Republic of Moldova, Romania and Tajikistan.

In April 2012 and under the auspices of the Danish EU Presidency, the Regional Office organized the European Diabetes Leadership Forum, with OECD and the Danish National Diabetes Association; and the First European Conference on Patient Empowerment, in relation to NCDs, with Danish health authorities, the Careum Foundation, Switzerland and the Expert Patient Programme, United Kingdom. In addition, the Regional Office provided information useful in policy-making, including a report on tools for intersectoral action on tobacco and nutrition in south-eastern Europe *(72)*.

Further, the Regional Office put together a package of supporting documents on the use of fiscal policies to prevent NCDs; it was used in a training seminar in Lithuania in September 2012 for health decision-makers from Albania, Bulgaria, Croatia, Estonia, Hungary, Lithuania, Poland, Slovakia and Ukraine. The Regional Office organized the seminar with the Countrywide Integrated Noncommunicable Diseases Intervention (CINDI) network, the University of Alberta, Canada and the Lithuanian University of Health Sciences.

Finally, the Regional Office held the WHO European Ministerial Conference on the Prevention and Control of Noncommunicable Diseases in the Context of Health 2020 in December 2013 in Ashgabat, Turkmenistan *(73)*. It asked health ministers in the WHO European Region to take stock of their achievements in the prevention and control of NCDs over the previous two years, and to declare their commitment to joint action in this area in the short and long terms. The participants comprised delegations from 35 European countries, international experts and representatives of partner and NGOs. Many countries explained how they were adapting their health systems to address the challenges of NCDs, working across sectors and developing appropriate health information systems, including: Azerbaijan, Belarus, Bosnia and Herzegovina, Bulgaria, Croatia, Georgia, Kazakhstan, Kyrgyzstan, Lithuania, the Republic of Moldova, Romania, Tajikistan and Ukraine. During the Conference, the Regional Office launched both its country assessment guide on strengthening health systems to secure better NCD outcomes and the *European tobacco control status report 2013 (74)*. The participants concluded their work by adopting the Ashgabat Declaration on the Prevention and Control

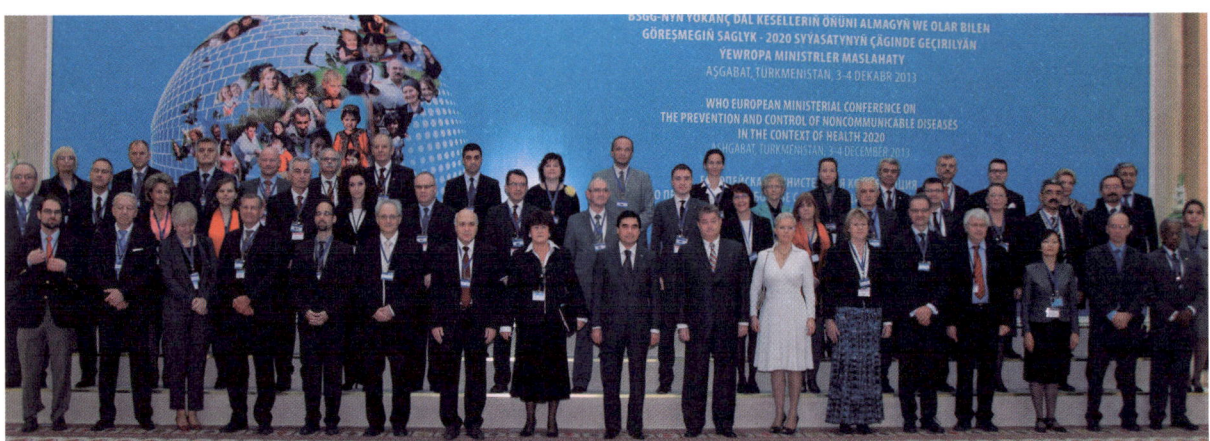

of Noncommunicable Diseases in the Context of Health 2020 (75), committing their countries to accelerate their efforts to fully implement the WHO Framework Convention on Tobacco Control (FCTC) with the shared ambition of ultimately making the WHO European Region tobacco free. The Declaration has three pillars: tobacco, acting across the whole of government and specific recommendations on accelerating the development of national targets.

Promoting healthy behaviour

Harmful alcohol use

To support action to reduce the harmful use of alcohol, the WHO Regional Office for Europe developed indicators and a checklist of action for policy-makers (76), and helped Member States – such as Belarus, Montenegro, the Republic of Moldova, the former Yugoslav Republic of Macedonia, and the Nordic and Baltic countries – update their alcohol policies, exchange ideas and take action.

Working closely with the EC on monitoring alcohol use, the Regional Office published a popular new book in March 2012: *Alcohol in the European Union. Consumption, harm and policy approaches* (77). In 2013 it issued Russian translations of major publications (76,78). With the health authorities in Poland and Turkey, the Regional Office held meetings of its national focal points for alcohol policy in 2012 and 2013, respectively, enabling them to exchange best practices and review new developments (79,80). It surveyed consumption, harm and policy responses in all 53 Member States and published the results for 35 countries (81).

Tobacco control

The Regional Office continued to support the ratification and implementation of the FCTC (82). It welcomed ratifications by the Czech Republic and Uzbekistan in 2012 and Tajikistan in 2013, which made the European Region the WHO region with the highest number of Parties, and a number of country initiatives. For example, Bulgaria, Hungary and Ukraine banned smoking in public places; France, Kazakhstan and the Russian Federation used pictorial health warnings on tobacco packaging; the Republic of Moldova adopted a strong five-year national action plan for tobacco control; Turkey celebrated a 4% decline in adult smoking prevalence between 2008 and 2012; Ukraine banned the advertising and promotion of tobacco products; and Uzbekistan strengthened its smoke-free legislation. Nevertheless, rates of implementation of the FCTC did not match the rate of ratification; the Ashgabat Declaration (75) could help countries correct this imbalance.

Supported by Switzerland, the Regional Office launched a new database on tobacco control legislation in the European Region that shows gaps and allows comparisons between countries (83). The WHO

Regional Director for Europe and the WHO Director-General pledged technical and political support to the proposed EU directive on tobacco products, and the Regional Office expressed its support by hosting a high-level meeting at the European Parliament on 30 May 2013 as part of the celebrations for World No Tobacco Day.

The themes for World No Tobacco Day 2012 and 2013 were the tobacco industry's interference in control efforts and banning tobacco advertising, promotion and sponsorship, respectively (84). As part of the celebrations, WHO gave awards to the prime ministers of Hungary and Kazakhstan, the Minister of Health of the Republic of Moldova and members of the parliaments of Ukraine and the United Kingdom, recognizing their strong commitment and whole-of-government approach to tobacco control.

Nutrition and physical activity

In March 2013, the WHO Regional Office for Europe held a meeting of nutrition focal points from 45 European Member States in Tel Aviv, Israel; the participants:

- reviewed their countries' progress in improving nutrition and physical activity, and implementing the European Charter on Counteracting Obesity and the WHO European Action Plan for Food and Nutrition Policy 2007–2012 (85,86);
- discussed the development of a new generation of policies on these topics, which could be the basis of a third food and nutrition action plan for the Region; and
- discussed building capacity for surveillance, monitoring and policy development in these areas, which would help to implement Health 2020 (11) and the NCD Action Plan (69).

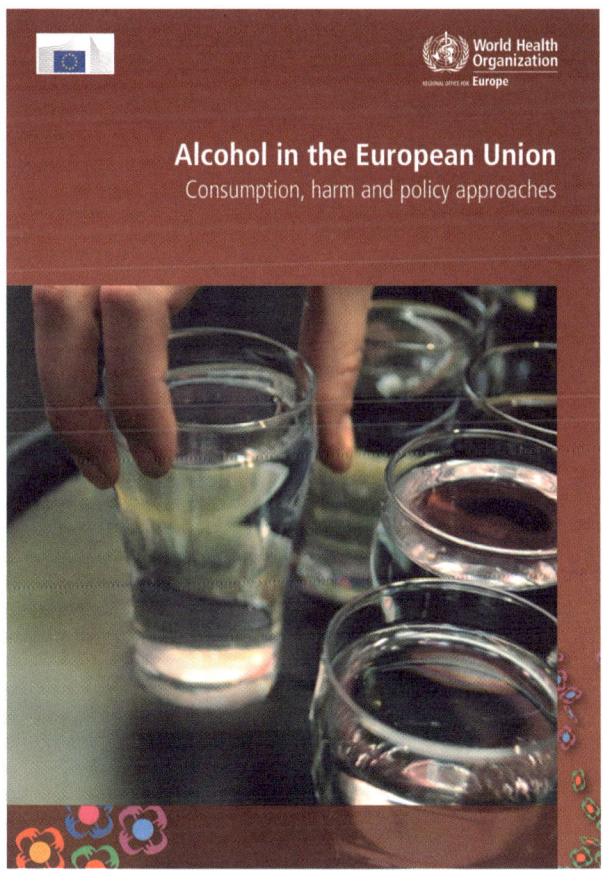

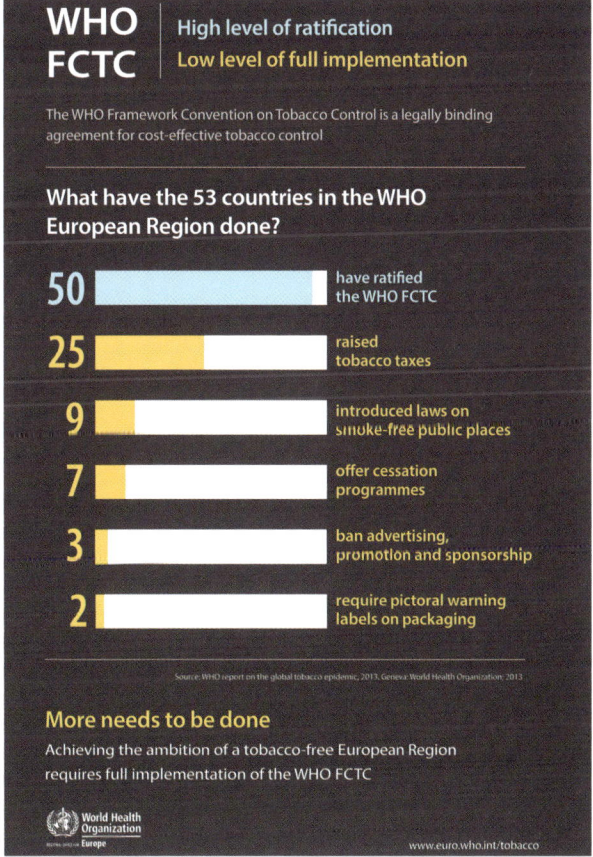

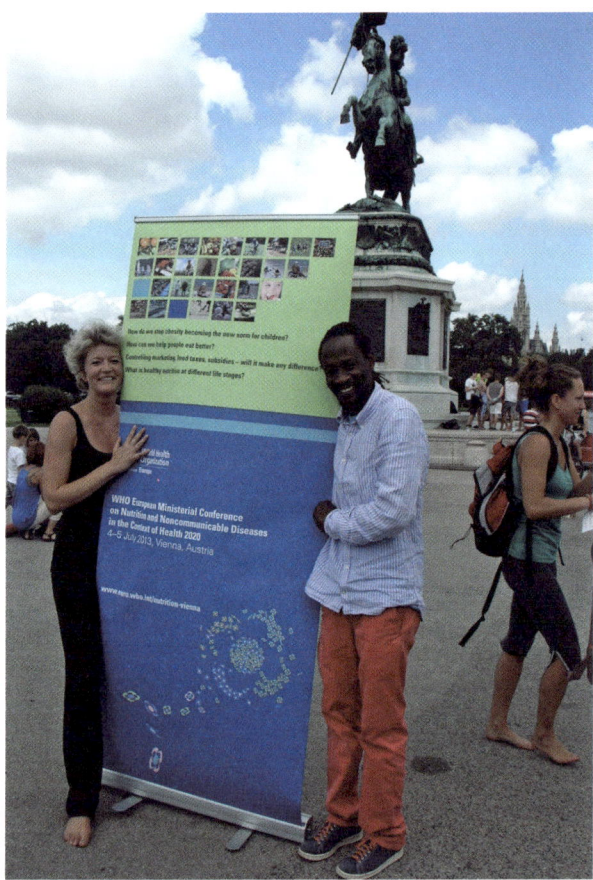

This was part of the preparations for the WHO European Ministerial Conference on Nutrition and Noncommunicable Diseases in the Context of Health 2020, held by the Regional Office in Vienna, Austria in July 2013 (87). Delegations from 47 European Member States, including 28 ministerial delegations, discussed coordinated action and cost-effective strategies on diet and physical activity in relation to NCDs and Health 2020. They described developments and policy interventions in their countries to address both nutrition and physical activity (in, for example, Finland, France, the Republic of Moldova, Slovenia, Ukraine and Uzbekistan) and childhood obesity (in, for example, Albania, Azerbaijan, Latvia, Malta and the Russian Federation). Following lengthy discussions, ministers signed the Vienna Declaration on Nutrition and Noncommunicable Diseases in the Context of Health 2020 (88), committing countries in the European Region to address the root causes of obesity and diet-related NCDs and to empower citizens to make healthy choices. The Declaration covers five priority areas:

- creating healthy food and drink environments and encouraging physical activity for all population groups;
- promoting the health gains of a healthy diet throughout the life-course, especially for the most vulnerable;
- reinforcing health systems to promote health and to provide services for NCDs;
- supporting surveillance, monitoring, evaluation and research of the population's nutritional status and behaviour; and
- strengthening governance, alliances and networks and empowering communities to engage in health promotion and prevention efforts.

Further, the Vienna Declaration urged the Regional Committee to mandate the development of a new action plan on food and nutrition and a strategy on physical activity. The 2013 Regional Committee agreed, endorsing the Declaration, calling on Member States to take action and asking the Regional Office to submit a new action plan and strategy to the 2015 and 2016 sessions, respectively (7).

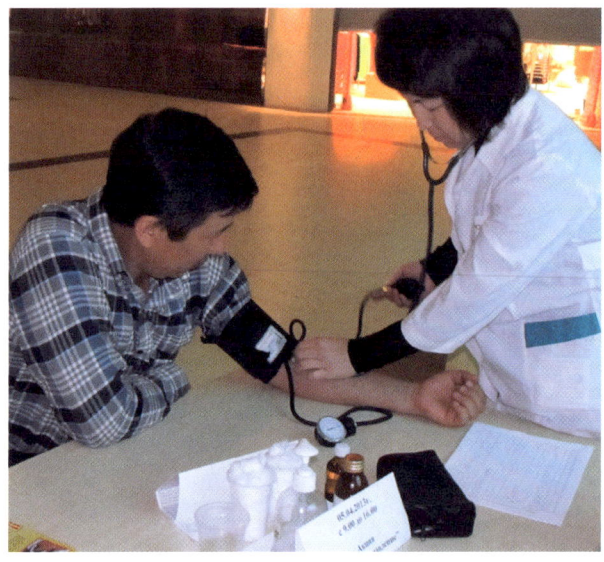

In addition, the WHO Regional Office for Europe focused on hypertension in celebrating World Health Day 2013 *(89)*. The wide range of activities conducted by Member States included several for prevention (in Croatia, Georgia, Kyrgyzstan, the Republic of Moldova and Uzbekistan), particularly through the reduction of dietary salt intake (in Estonia, Hungary, Montenegro and Turkey).

Work on physical activity included the publication of guidance on promoting such activity in socially disadvantaged groups and young people *(90,91)*.

Mental health

The Regional Office carried out a two-year consultative process to develop a European action plan on mental health for submission to the 2013 Regional Committee. Member States warmly welcomed the European Mental Health Action Plan *(92)*, and commended its timeliness in the light of the economic crisis *(7)*. The Action Plan covers 2014–2020, is linked to Health 2020 *(11)* and has seven objectives to ensure:

- equal opportunities to mental well-being throughout life;
- human rights for those with mental health problems;
- accessible and affordable mental health services, with priority on community care;
- respectful, safe and effective treatment;
- health systems that provide good physical and mental health for all;
- mental health systems that are coordinated with other systems and partners; and
- governance and delivery of mental health systems based on sound information and knowledge *(92)*.

In addition, the Regional Office supported the development and implementation of community-based services in Turkey for people with mental health problems and intellectual disabilities, co-funded by an EU grant. It supported the drafting of policies and delivery of services in countries including Azerbaijan, Georgia, Kyrgyzstan, the Republic of Moldova and Tajikistan.

Violence and injury prevention

The Regional Office's work to prevent violence and injury included efforts to improve road safety and tackle the abuse of children and women. Work to improve road safety, particularly for vulnerable road users such as children and elderly people, included surveying measures taken by 51 countries *(93)* and taking part in campaigns such as the Second United Nations Global Road Safety Week in May 2013, which focused on pedestrian safety.

The Regional Office surveyed maltreatment and other adverse experiences in childhood and held policy dialogues on them in several countries. It published a report *(94)*, launched during the 2013 Regional Committee, detailing the types and extent of maltreatment of children in Europe, the benefits of prevention for health in later life and the value of targeted prevention initiatives for those most at risk.

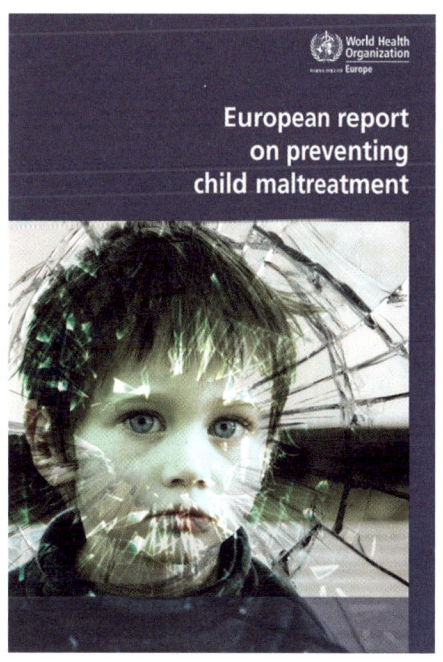

In connection with the United Nations International Day for the Elimination of Violence against Women, 25 November 2013, the Regional Office, the European Institute for Gender Equality and the City of Vienna held a large meeting to discuss intersectoral strategies to combat the problem. The participants comprised more than 200 representatives from 53 countries.

Promoting health throughout the life-course

Maternal, child and adolescent health and well-being

The Regional Office's efforts to improve the health and well-being of mothers, children and adolescents included a life-course approach with a focus on prevention, health promotion and the quality of care. For example, it organized a regional meeting to improve access to reproductive health services, including safe abortion, in Riga, Latvia in May 2012. Co-hosted by the International Planned Parenthood Federation European Network, a long-term partner, the meeting attracted 100 participants from more than 30 countries and 15 international organizations. In addition, the Regional Office held a meeting in October 2013 to report the results of a project to reduce maternal and neonatal morbidity and mortality in Armenia and Kyrgyzstan by improving primary health care for women and babies, and referral systems during pregnancy and after childbirth. The project was financed and implemented by the Government of the Russian Federation.

The Regional Office also took part – with technical experts and representatives of United Nations agencies (including UNFPA), governments and NGOs from all six WHO regions – in global efforts to reduce the harm to health resulting from child marriage, which occurs in some eastern countries in the Region *(95,96)*. In December 2012, the Regional Office and the UNFPA Eastern Europe and Central Asia Regional Office agreed to further strengthen their technical, strategic and policy collaboration, which would include cooperation on the post-2015 development agenda *(97)*. The agreement signed between the two in 2013 *(7)* is described in Chapter 1.

In addition, the Regional Office supported countries – such as Albania, Armenia, Azerbaijan, Kyrgyzstan, the Republic of Moldova, the Russian Federation, Tajikistan, Turkmenistan and Uzbekistan – in improving care and services for children and adolescents in 2012–2013. It also published the latest international report of the Health Behaviour in School-aged Children (HBSC) study *(98)* in English and Russian, which provides a systematic statistical base for describing cross-national patterns in young people's health and well-being *(99)*. Decision-makers throughout the Region warmly welcomed the report, and it won a prize in the 2013 British Medical Association (BMA) Medical Book Awards competition.

Healthy ageing

The centrepiece of the Regional Office's work for healthy ageing was the development of the strategy and action plan for healthy ageing in Europe, which the Regional Committee adopted in 2012 *(6,100)*. With clear links to Health 2020, it contains four strategic priority areas for action: healthy ageing over the life-course, supportive environments, people-centred health and long-term care systems fit for ageing populations, and strengthening of the evidence base and research. The drafting process, in which representatives of the EC participated, included work to ensure that the strategy and action plan complemented measures taken by other partners in Europe, such as OECD and UNECE.

In addition, the Regional Office organized and contributed to a series of events across the European Region to celebrate World Health Day 2012, whose theme was "active ageing" *(89)*. These included a regional launch, with officials from Denmark and Italy *(101)*. Partners in such work included the EU, which designated 2012 as the European Year for Active Ageing and Solidarity between Generations.

Late in 2013, the Regional Office and the EC Directorate-General for Employment, Social Affairs and Inclusion started a joint two-year project for age-friendly environments in Europe. Its goals are:

- to provide tools to help local policy-makers identify priority areas for action, design local action plans and plan the evaluation and monitoring of age-friendly policies;
- to identify and disseminate good practices and connect relevant initiatives, projects and developments for age-friendly cities; and
- to strengthen the networks of cities, communities and regions active in the field and create guidance that helps implement intersectoral action and policies for healthy ageing.

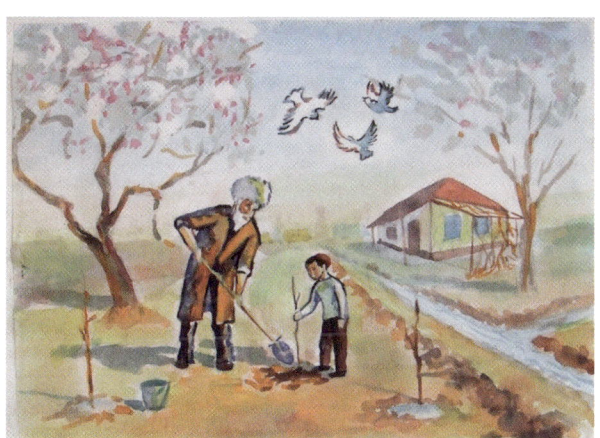

4. COMMUNICABLE DISEASES

In its work on communicable diseases, the WHO Regional Office for Europe focused on unfinished business: implementing action plans on three problems placing a significant burden on public health in Europe; pursuing or maintaining the eradication of polio, malaria and measles/rubella; and fighting vaccine-preventable infections by promoting immunization. It also started to address new business: the threat of re-emerging vector-borne disease.

Implementing action plans

Once the 2011 Regional Committee adopted action plans on multidrug- and extensively drug-resistant TB (M/XDR-TB), HIV/AIDS and antibiotic resistance *(102–104)*, the Regional Office and its partners started implementing them. In deepening partnership with the EU, the Regional Office held live Twitter chats with the European Centre for Disease Prevention and Control (ECDC) to mark World TB Day, European Antibiotic Awareness Day and World AIDS Day, as well as issuing annual joint reports on TB and AIDS surveillance in Europe (*105–108)*.

M/XDR-TB

Working closely with the Global Fund to Fight AIDS, Tuberculosis and Malaria, the EC and ECDC, the Regional Office reviewed programmes on TB and M/XDR-TB in, for example, Azerbaijan, Belarus, Bosnia and Herzegovina, Hungary, Kazakhstan, Latvia, the Netherlands, the Republic of Moldova, Slovakia, Tajikistan and Ukraine, along with Kosovo (in accordance with Security Council resolution 1244 (1999)). With partners such as the Green Light Committee, the Regional Office supported countries such as Belarus, Portugal, Romania, Tajikistan, Turkmenistan and Uzbekistan in taking action to improve care and other services, and helped countries such as Armenia, Belarus, Switzerland, Turkmenistan and Ukraine to make or update policies and action plans in line with the European action plan. The Regional Office hosted a "Faces of Tuberculosis" photo exhibition at the European Parliament for World TB Day in March 2013; in return, 14 members of the European Parliament, from six political groups and 10 countries, launched a written declaration to the WHO European Region in the Parliament in April, calling on the EC to support the Regional Office's roadmap and action plan on M/XDR-TB *(102)*.

The Regional Office held regional workshops in October and November 2013 to support the implementation of the action plan, addressing: anti-TB drug resistance, ethical and human rights issues in preventing and treating M/XDR-TB, results-based management approaches and models of care. In the last of these, participants discussed four best practices in providing patient-centred care of TB and MDR-TB patients from the Regional Office's recently published compendium *(109)* to identify improvements they could make in their countries.

HIV/AIDS

In response to the rising number of people living with HIV, the European Action Plan for HIV/AIDS *(103)* was implemented at full speed, offering a framework for urgent action and accelerating effective responses by strengthening health systems. In 2012–2013, the Regional Office provided useful information, such as revised care protocols and profiles of the situation in countries *(110–111)*. With a range of partners, including the Joint United Nations Programme on HIV/AIDS (UNAIDS) and its cosponsors (including the United Nations Office on Drugs and Crime (UNODC), the World Bank, UNICEF, UNFPA and UNDP) and ECDC, it supported work to improve care services, particularly those for injecting drug users and other key vulnerable populations living with HIV, in countries such as Belarus, Estonia, Greece, Kazakhstan, Kyrgyzstan, Portugal, the Russian Federation, Tajikistan, Ukraine and Uzbekistan.

During 2012–2013, the Regional Office visited countries to monitor progress in the elimination of mother-to-child transmission of both HIV and syphilis, in collaboration with UNICEF, UNAIDS and UNFPA. It also evaluated collaborative activities and integration of services for HIV and TB in seven countries (Azerbaijan, Belarus, Kazakhstan, Kyrgyzstan, Tajikistan, Ukraine and Uzbekistan), and recommended increasing access to testing, diagnosis, treatment and monitoring for coinfected patients.

In October 2013, the Regional Office held a technical consultation in Turkey on expanding the eligibility criteria for antiretroviral treatment and implementing the new WHO guidelines on this topic *(112)*. The participants comprised representatives of 13 Member States (Armenia, Azerbaijan, Belarus, Georgia, Kazakhstan, Kyrgyzstan, the Republic of Moldova, the Russian Federation, Tajikistan, Turkey, Turkmenistan, Ukraine and Uzbekistan), national experts in HIV/AIDS, and representatives of civil-society organizations and partner organizations (UNAIDS, UNICEF, the Global Fund and the United States Centers for Disease Control and Prevention (CDC)). The participants made plans to implement new WHO guidelines *(112)* in their countries and called for support from WHO in this task. In addition, the Regional Office designated new WHO collaborating centres in Denmark and Lithuania on HIV and viral hepatitis, and on reduction of the harm done by drug use, respectively, in the second half of 2013.

Antibiotic resistance

The Regional Office implemented the European strategic action plan on antibiotic resistance *(104)* with Member States and a broad coalition of other partners. Initial work focused on national coordination and surveillance; it included an agreement with RIVM and the European Society of Clinical Microbiology and Infectious Diseases (ESCMID) to expand surveillance of antimicrobial resistance to cover all countries in the WHO European Region. The new Central Asia and Eastern European Surveillance of Antimicrobial Resistance (CAESAR) network is a key component of the action plan *(104)*. In cooperation with RIVM, ESCMID, and the University of Antwerp, Belgium, the Regional Office also organized, for example, intercountry workshops on the rational use of antibiotics, a workshop on surveillance of antimicrobial use and resistance, and awareness campaigns for experts from over a dozen southern and eastern non-European countries. The Regional Office worked closely with ECDC to ensure compatible and complementary data collection.

Similarly, the Regional Office worked with ECDC to expand European Antibiotic Awareness Day 2012 from the EU to the whole European Region. The Patron of the Regional Office, HRH Crown Princess Mary of Denmark, made a statement to mark the Day, as well as addressing a conference on antimicrobial resistance held by Denmark during its EU Presidency. The Regional Office supported activities to mark European Antibiotic Awareness Day 2012 and 2013 in more than 10 countries outside the EU, including Georgia, Kyrgyzstan, Montenegro and the former Yugoslav Republic of Macedonia. Finally, the Regional Office supported Member States in developing national strategic action plans on antimicrobial resistance with intersectoral coordination.

Eliminating diseases

In 2012–2013, the WHO Regional Office for Europe supported the maintenance of Europe's polio-free status, its continued progress against malaria and its struggle against measles and rubella.

Polio

Meeting in June 2012, the European Regional Certification Commission for Poliomyelitis Eradication (RCC) confirmed that the European Region remained polio free, but urged Member States to maintain high immunization coverage and effective surveillance until global eradication is achieved *(113)*. This was the prelude to the Regional Office's celebration of the tenth anniversary of the European Region's certification as polio free, on 21 June. The Regional Office used World Polio Day, in October 2012, to urge countries to maintain their momentum on immunization against this crippling and potentially deadly disease. The Regional Office regularly published information from surveillance of acute flaccid paralysis, along with epidemiological data on measles and rubella *(114)*.

In May 2013, the RCC reaffirmed the Region's polio-free status and identified some areas at higher risk should wild poliovirus be introduced. Later in the year, the Regional Office supported immunization campaigns in Israel (after the detection of wild poliovirus 1 in sewage samples) and Turkey (as part of the cross-regional response to a polio outbreak in the Syrian Arab Republic) *(114)*. With USAID and the Ministry of Health of Tajikistan, the Regional Office

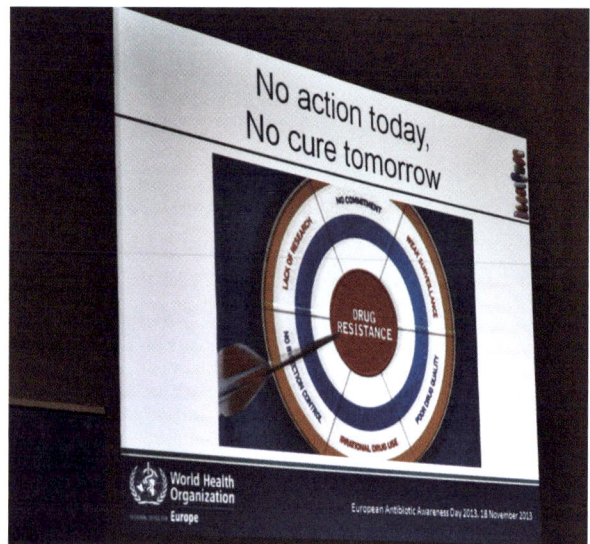

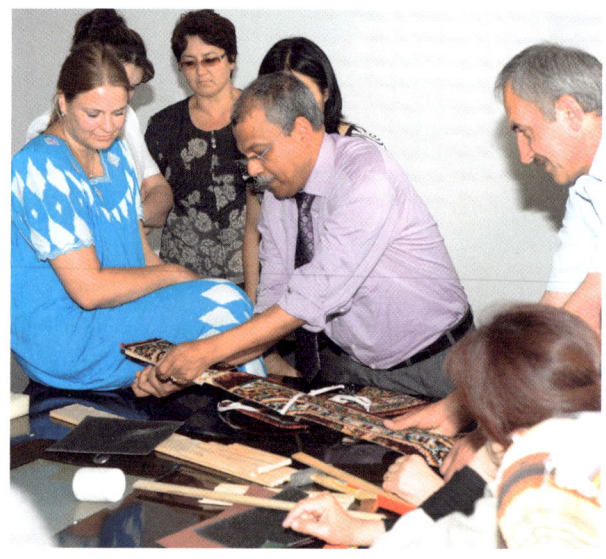

Communicable diseases

started a three-year project to improve services for disabled survivors of the 2010 polio outbreak. Looking towards the final eradication of polio and building on WHO's Global Vaccine Action Plan, the Regional Office proposed to produce an updated regional plan that would be harmonized with the Health 2020 policy, respond to regional and national needs, and contain tailored regional targets. It would consult with Member States, and present the draft regional vaccine action plan to the Regional Committee in 2014 *(7)*.

Malaria

The Region continued its progress towards eliminating malaria by 2015. Only five countries reported malaria cases: Azerbaijan, Georgia, Tajikistan, Turkey and (with a small outbreak in 2011) Greece. WHO certified Kazakhstan malaria free in 2012. Through World Malaria Day 2012 and with partners including the Global Fund to Fight AIDS, Tuberculosis and Malaria, the Bill & Melinda Gates Foundation and the Russian Federation, the Regional Office supported Armenia and Turkmenistan in working to maintain their malaria-free status. The Regional Office held a meeting to synchronize elimination activities in Tajikistan and Afghanistan in May 2012. After malaria cases increased in 2012 (253 cases were reported in the five affected countries), the Regional Office called on affected countries to sustain malaria interventions, even in times of economic austerity, on World Malaria Day 2013. With WHO headquarters and host governments, in summer 2013 the Regional Office held training courses on malaria elimination and certification in Azerbaijan and Turkmenistan for specialists from Azerbaijan, Georgia, Kyrgyzstan, Tajikistan and Uzbekistan. Tajikistan continued to work towards certification as malaria free, and Kyrgyzstan and Uzbekistan hoped to begin the process at the end of 2013.

In work on both polio and malaria, the Russian Federation and Turkey provided valuable financial and technical support, and the Regional Office worked closely with the WHO Eastern Mediterranean Region.

Measles and rubella

Unfortunately, large outbreaks of measles and rubella imperilled the Region's goal of eliminating measles and rubella by 2015. Surveillance by the Regional Office and ECDC revealed that rubella cases increased steeply in 2012, and there were over 20 000 measles cases in the first six months of 2013 *(114,115)*. In response to the situation, the Regional Office presented a package of accelerated action to eliminate the two diseases *(116)* to the Regional Committee in September; it has six components: strengthening of vaccination and immunization systems; surveillance; outbreak preparedness and response; communications, information and advocacy; resource mobilization and partnerships; and verification of measles and rubella elimination. In addition, cross-border and interregional coordination would be strengthened, particularly with the WHO Eastern Mediterranean Region. The Regional Committee welcomed the package *(7)* and, one month later, the European Technical Advisory Group of Experts on Immunization called on Member States to make or revisit their action plans for measles and rubella elimination and urgently to address immunity gaps in their populations.

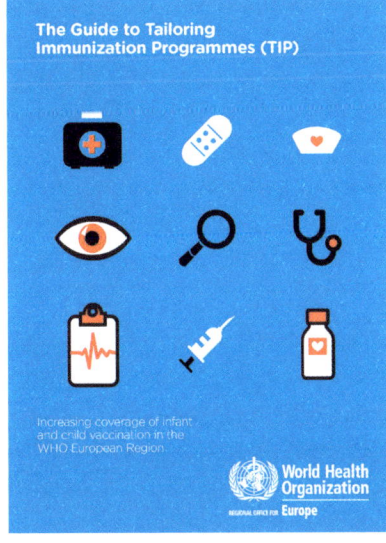

The Regional Office supported countries' work to reach susceptible populations, and provided strong political support and sustained funding for immunization programmes. For example, it developed an innovative toolkit, pilot-tested in Bulgaria and then published in connection with European Immunization Week 2013 *(117)*, to help countries understand what influences vaccination among at-risk and vulnerable groups. It also sought to strengthen laboratory surveillance, for example, by holding a joint meeting for the national and subnational reference laboratories in the Russian Federation and other newly independent states (NIS) in March 2012, with the support of the Institute of Immunology of Luxembourg. In September 2013, it published new guidelines to support rapid response to measles and rubella outbreaks *(118)*.

In addition, the Regional Office began to document progress towards eradication by developing a framework for the verification process and convening independent experts to serve on the European Regional Verification Commission for Measles and Rubella Elimination (RVC). RVC accepted the framework at its first meeting in January 2012, and urged countries to form their own national verification commissions and use a standard template for their reports. With ECDC, the Regional Office supported this process by holding meetings of the RVC with commissions and focal points from groups of countries: 12 NIS (October 2012, Uzbekistan), 16 northern and western countries (January 2013, Denmark) and central and south-eastern countries (February 2013, Bulgaria).

Promoting immunization

The WHO Regional Office for Europe promotes immunization, the most effective instrument against vaccine-preventable diseases, particularly through European Immunization Week *(119)*, held in April each year. The 2012 and 2013 sessions of the Week were the most successful yet, taking place as part of World Immunization Week and involving all 53 countries in the European Region, which conducted national and local initiatives to raise awareness and increase vaccination uptake.

To help countries, health systems and service providers to be strong advocates for immunization, the Regional Office provided key messages for each Week, and resources such as the online Immunization Resource Centre for health workers, a guide to tailoring immunization programmes and a generic app code that countries could tailor quickly and cheaply into a simple telephone-based tool to remind parents when their children's vaccinations are due *(117,120)*. The Regional Office, countries and partners – such as the GAVI Alliance, the Bill & Melinda Gates Foundation, the Measles & Rubella Initiative, Shot@Life, ECDC, UNICEF and the European Confederation of Primary Care Paediatricians – worked hard to spread the message, writing articles, producing videos, using social media such as Twitter and carrying out a wide range of other activities. HRH Princess Mathilde (now HM Queen Mathilde) of Belgium, WHO's Special

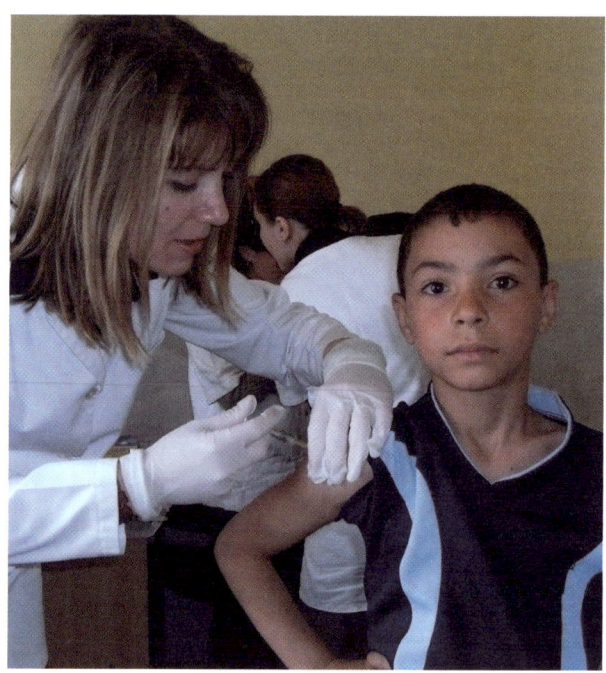

Representative for Immunization, stressed the vital role played by front-line health workers in national immunization programmes in 2012, and HRH Crown Princess Mary of Denmark continued her support for the initiative by making statements in both 2012 and 2013. In both years, the Week received tremendous media coverage, sending the message on the importance of immunization throughout the Region.

Similarly, the Regional Office established an influenza awareness day – held in November 2012 and 2013 just before the start of the influenza season – to promote seasonal influenza vaccination, focusing on key groups such as health care workers and the elderly *(121)*.

the Regional Office worked to raise awareness of the problem, with ECDC, EMCA and the European Network for Arthropod Vector Surveillance for Human Public Health (VBORNET).

The Regional Office also worked to map the extent of leishmaniasis in Europe, holding a subregional meeting on leishmaniasis control in Georgia, in April 2013, and to help countries secure supplies of deworming tablets to protect children against soil-transmitted helminthiasis. Supported by the Rostropovich–Vishnevskaya Foundation, the Regional Office and the Government of Tajikistan conducted a campaign to treat people infected by worms in autumn 2013.

Re-emerging vector-borne and parasitic diseases

Vector-borne and parasitic diseases arouse increasing concern in the European Region. Mosquito vector activity is a growing problem, driven mostly by the globalization of travel and trade, urbanization and climate change. In cooperation with WHO headquarters, ECDC, the European Mosquito Control Association (EMCA) and Member States, the Regional Office developed a regional framework for action in this area and presented it to the 2013 Regional Committee *(122)*. It lists essential actions for countries that face problems related to invasive mosquito vectors, including dengue and chikungunya fever, and provides a platform to facilitate interaction between countries, including across borders. The Regional Committee supported the framework and urged Member States to use it as guidance in developing national action plans *(7)*. In addition,

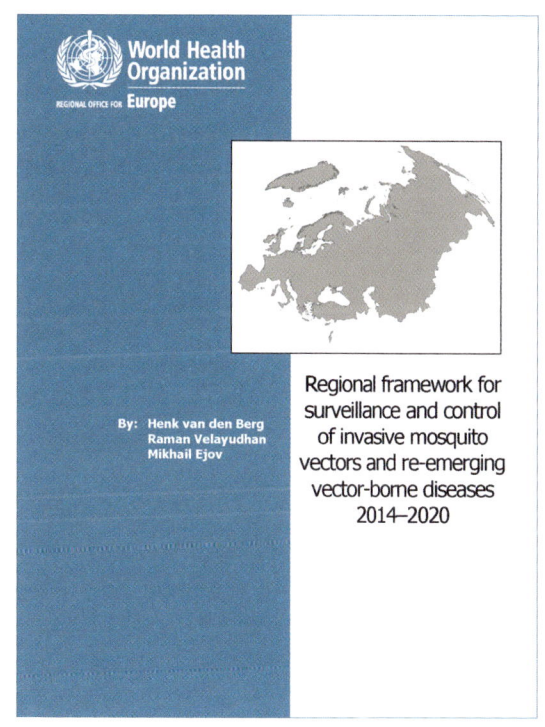

5. PREPAREDNESS, SURVEILLANCE AND RESPONSE

In line with its role as a leader in humanitarian and public health emergencies, the WHO Regional Office for Europe worked to help countries prepare for and cope with emergencies and health crises, in close collaboration with WHO headquarters and the EC and its institutions. The 2013 Regional Committee agreed to expand the Regional Office's capacity to support Member States by accepting the Government of Turkey's offer to host a new GDO for preparedness for humanitarian and health emergencies (7).

Preparedness for emergencies and disasters

International Health Regulations

Under the International Health Regulations (IHR) (123), the European Region has a well established system, including an active network of national focal points, for vigorous monitoring of events that may threaten public health. The Regional Office assessed and documented over 700 public health events in the Region, often consulting the affected Member States through IHR channels. In 2012–2013, for example, the Regional Office monitored imported and secondary cases of Middle East respiratory syndrome coronavirus (MERS-CoV) in France, Germany, Italy and the United Kingdom, gathering and sharing detailed information about each case through confidential IHR mechanisms; strengthened surveillance for MERS-CoV and possible human infections with the avian influenza A(H7N9) virus that emerged in China; and closely followed a dengue outbreak in Portugal.

The Regional Office supported countries in implementing the IHR through training to build core capacities, for example, in ship sanitation inspectors in Estonia, with the Estonian Health Board; and in Balkan countries, in collaboration with the Health Protection Agency (HPA) of the United Kingdom. In 2012 it launched the "Better Labs for Better Health" initiative in eastern European countries to improve the quality of laboratory services, promote better use of existing resources and increase preparedness for emerging diseases. In October 2013, the Regional Office and partners organized meetings to increase countries' core capacities in surveillance and response and at points of entry. The meeting in Denmark organized with the International Committee of Military Medicine (ICMM) concluded that countries' military health services should take part in their efforts to comply with the IHR. A biregional multicountry expert workshop in Kazakhstan to strengthen the capacity requirements for the IHR at ground crossings was organized with the WHO Regional Office for the

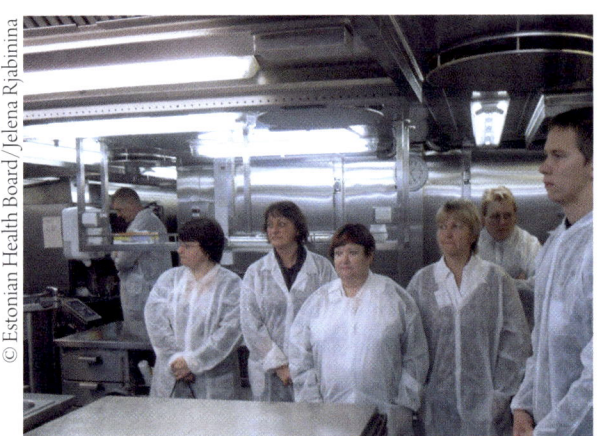
© Estonian Health Board/Jelena Rjabinina

Western Pacific, and brought together national focal points for the IHR and experts working in the area from Belarus, China, Kazakhstan, Kyrgyzstan, the Russian Federation and Ukraine.

In February 2013, with support from the EC, Germany, the United Kingdom and WHO headquarters, the Regional Office held a meeting in Luxembourg, at which national focal points from 50 European States Parties took stock of the implementation process five years after the IHR's entry into force, called for this process to include action by a range of sectors and partners, and asked WHO to assist countries in testing existing mechanisms. As many countries still lacked core capacities for IHR implementation in 2013, WHO asked its regional committees to propose criteria for granting extensions. The WHO Regional Office for Europe proposed to the Regional Committee for Europe that countries apply to the WHO Director-General in writing, explaining the circumstances and including an implementation plan *(7)*. It reported Member States' reactions at and after the discussion to the Director-General, for submission to the WHO Executive Board in January 2014.

Preparedness

The Regional Office intensified its support to Member States in strengthening their capacities to prepare for emergencies *(124)*. It continued its assessments of health systems' preparedness *(125)*, and published a two-part toolkit for assessing capacity for crisis management, the results of a joint project supported by the EC *(126,127)*. It analysed hospital vulnerability in countries such as Montenegro, and supported the development and implementation of action plans for improvement. The Regional Office also supported projects to increase hospital preparedness and resilience in the Republic of Moldova, Tajikistan and the former Yugoslav Republic of Macedonia, and conducted training workshops in Israel to build capacity in public health and emergency management in countries including Albania, Azerbaijan, the Czech Republic, Georgia, Kyrgyzstan, Poland, the Republic of Moldova and Ukraine. In addition, the Regional Office held workshops on pandemic preparedness for 23 countries across the Region in 2012 and for 40 countries in 2013.

Further, the Regional Office revised its emergency procedures and tested them in exercises, and made the emergency operations centre at its new premises fully operational, as the new global WHO Emergency Response Framework *(128)* foresees a greater role for regional and country offices (see below). Her Majesty Queen Margrethe II of Denmark, Prime Minister Helle Thorning-Schmidt of Denmark and United Nations Secretary-General Ban Ki-moon visited the operations centre in July 2013.

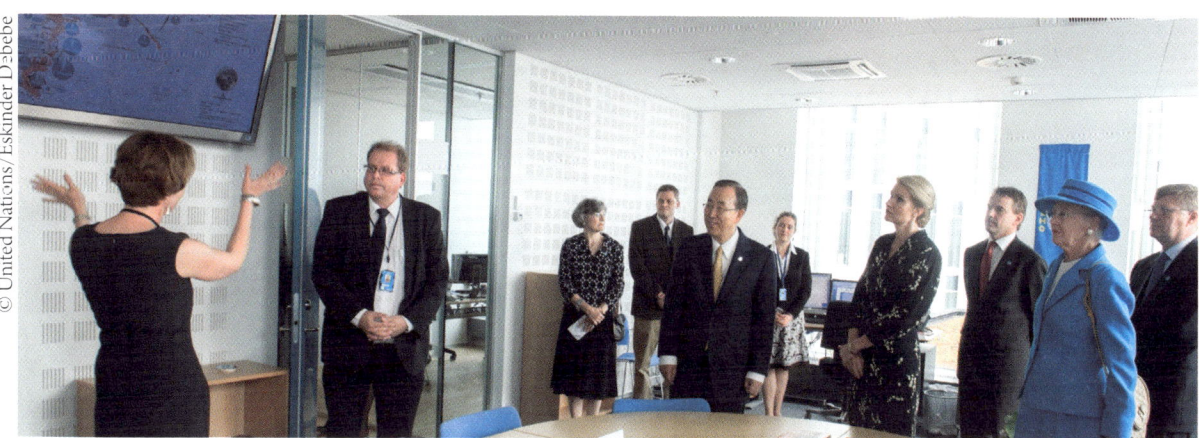

Mass gatherings

Work with partners and national authorities to anticipate and prepare for the health needs associated with mass gatherings in the Region was an evolving priority *(129)*. With governments, ECDC and WHO headquarters, the Regional Office established an enhanced monitoring system in this new area for use during the European football championship, hosted by Poland and Ukraine, and the Olympic and Paralympic Games, hosted by the United Kingdom in 2012. The Regional Office and HPA cooperated to provide health advice to physicians for teams taking part in these events, as well as producing guidance for travellers.

This work can not only prevent health problems at mass gatherings but also leave a valuable legacy: a sustainable positive impact on public health systems and a contribution to implementing the IHR *(123)*. With WHO headquarters, ECDC and WHO collaborating centres in Serbia and the United Kingdom, the Regional Office used the lessons learnt in 2012 to help build capacity in managing the risks of communicable diseases during mass gatherings in Slovenia, which hosted the European basketball championship in September 2013. With ECDC and the Slovenian National Institute of Public Health, the Regional Office published health advice to travellers attending the event *(129)*.

Surveillance

The Regional Office does much of its work on disease surveillance with ECDC, as described in Chapter 4. It also coordinates the surveillance of influenza with ECDC, and publishes a weekly bulletin in English and Russian *(130)* that includes data from 47 of the Region's 53 Member States, as well as reports describing the key features of the 2011/2012 and 2012/2013 influenza seasons. The bulletin describes the timing, spread, severity and impact of the influenza season and thus informs national prevention and control measures. With ECDC, the Regional Office held annual meetings on influenza surveillance in 2012 and 2013.

Responses to emergencies and disasters

In addition to tracking large numbers of emergencies in the European Region, the Regional Office helped countries respond to several major public health emergencies and disasters in 2012–2013 through various missions and investigations *(37,124)*. For example, Regional Office staff visited Krymsk, in the southern part of the Russian Federation, to offer assistance in recovery from floods in July 2012, and in December – with representatives of the Office of the United Nations High Commissioner for Refugees (UNHCR), UNICEF, UNFPA and IOM – formed

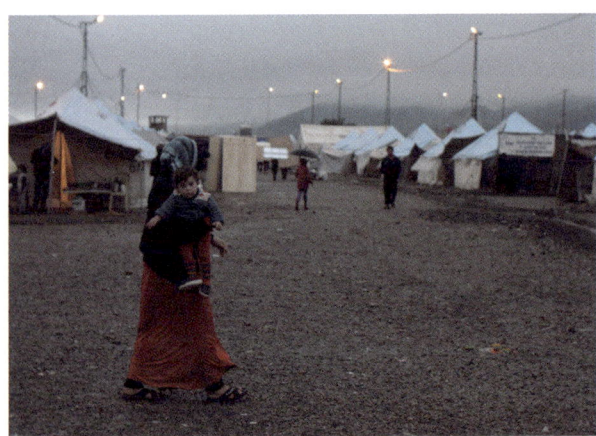
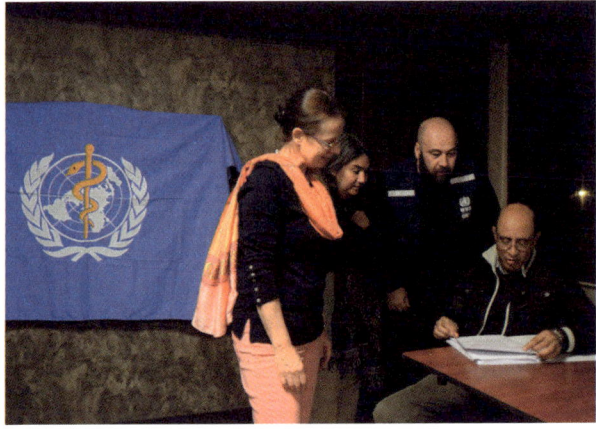

part of a joint United Nations health mission visiting four camps set up in Turkey for refugees from the conflict in the Syrian Arab Republic. Supported by the Turkish health and other authorities, the mission commended the Turkish Government's extensive efforts and began to develop possible options for joint projects to support them. WHO established a field presence in Gaziantep, Turkey in October 2013, to work with Turkish authorities in addressing the evolving health needs of Syrian refugees. It coordinated health partners providing services to Syrians in southern Turkey, and supported, for example, the immunization campaign against polio described in Chapter 4.

The Regional Office also sent experts outside the WHO European Region to support the global WHO response to three grade III emergencies under the WHO Emergency Response Framework *(128)*: to Jordan to support the global response to the crisis in the Syrian Arab Republic, the Philippines to support relief efforts following typhoon Haiyan and the Central African Republic to strengthen the WHO country team.

6. EUROPEAN ENVIRONMENT AND HEALTH PROCESS

In 2012–2013, the Regional Office scaled up its technical work on environment and health *(131)* to achieve the commitments in the Parma Declaration *(132)* within the framework of the European environment and health process, and the European Environment and Health Ministerial Board led the process with a stronger mandate for intersectoral governance *(133)*.

Governance

At its third meeting, in Azerbaijan in November 2012, the Board continued work to determine key priorities in the European environment and health process until 2016, in the context of Health 2020, and delivered discussion points on the need to integrate health arguments into the outcome document of Rio+20 (the United Nations Conference on Sustainable Development). It also agreed that an environment and health gateway, an online knowledge repository and information portal, would be developed to provide countries with resources to take action on environment and health priorities. At its fourth meeting, in Serbia in April 2013, the Board:

- completed its reports to the WHO Regional Committee for Europe *(134)* and the UNECE Committee on Environmental Policy, analysing the main experiences of its first three years; and
- called for the scaling up of work on air quality and the elimination of asbestos-related diseases, and the implementation of multilateral environmental agreements relevant to health, encouraging Member States to sign and ratify those to which they had not already acceded *(133)*.

The 2013 Regional Committee welcomed the Board's report, emphasized the importance of the environment and health process to achieving the

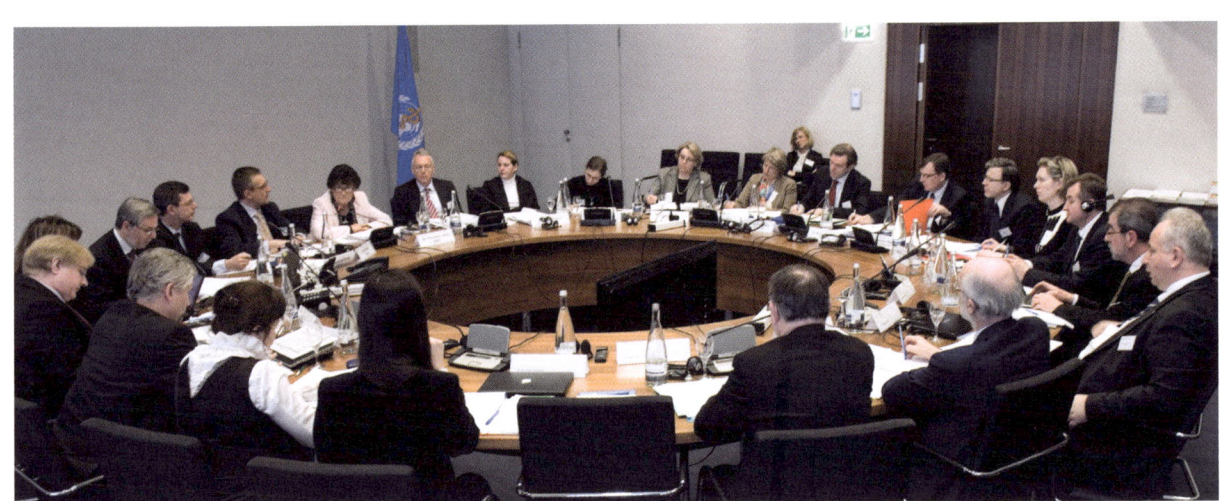

goals of Health 2020 *(11)* and selected new members of the Board: Croatia and Georgia for a two-year term of office (2014–2015) and Lithuania and Spain for a three-year term of office (2014–2016), exceptionally, to ensure continuity by staggering changes in membership *(7)*.

Meeting in the Netherlands in June 2012, the European Environment and Health Task Force agreed to monitor progress towards the Parma targets *(135)*. At its third meeting in Belgium in December 2013, the Task Force approved a workplan for 2014 that focused on preparing a review of progress in meeting the commitments in the Parma Declaration *(132)*. The review would take place midway between the 2010 Fifth Ministerial Conference on Environment and Health, in Parma, Italy, and the sixth conference, planned for 2016. Participants representing 30 countries agreed to scale up action to free Europe from asbestos-related diseases and exposure to second-hand tobacco smoke and toxic chemicals by 2015, and to provide every child in Europe with access to safe water and sanitation, and healthy and safe environments in which to be physically active by 2020.

Technical work

An agreement with the German Government, signed in February 2012, enabled the Regional Office to consolidate its environment and health programmes in Bonn. Technical work addressed a wide range of topics, such as implementing the WHO global plan of action for workers' health *(136)*. To support the elimination of asbestos-related diseases, the Regional Office held a meeting in Germany in November 2012 to help European countries quantify the human and financial burden of these diseases by using a WHO–ILO (International Labour Organization) outline to prepare national profiles. A workshop for 100 experts and European country representatives, held in Germany in October 2013, reviewed scientific and policy approaches to health effects from exposure to multiple risk factors, with special focus on asbestos, chemicals, air quality and housing *(131)*.

The activities to address the impact of climate change on health included:

- completing and disseminating the results of a project to strengthen health systems' capacity to respond to the health effects of climate change in seven countries: Albania, Kazakhstan, Kyrgyzstan, the Russian Federation, Tajikistan, the former Yugoslav Republic of Macedonia and Uzbekistan *(137)*;
- contributing the results of the Regional Office project on climate, environment and health action plan and information system (CEHAPIS) to underpin the health component of the new EU policy on climate change *(138)*;
- reviewing new evidence of the health impact of air quality, with funding from the EC, indicating the need to revise the WHO air quality guidelines and policies in Member States *(139–141)*;
- developing an economic analysis tool to support adaptation planning in Member States *(142)*; and
- helping to strengthen health systems to deal with the health effects of climate change.

The Regional Office also issued advice to health care professionals and the public on protecting health from the effects of extreme heat and cold.

Work for food safety included workshops and training – in collaboration with partners such as the Food and Agriculture Organization of the United Nations (FAO), the European Food Safety Authority (EFSA) and ECDC – on integrated surveillance, the prevention and control of foodborne diseases, Codex Alimentarius, food safety risk communication, and antibiotic resistance from a food safety perspective. In addition, the Regional Office provided countries with technical support during food-safety emergencies.

The Regional Office worked closely with UNECE to support the implementation of multilateral environmental agreements such as the Protocol on Water and Health, co-convening the third session of the Meeting of the Parties in 2013. Further, WHO-led networks were established in the European Region on chemical safety and economics, environment and health. The Regional Office published a report on how to incorporate economics into evidence-based decision-making in environment and health, including a draft strategic framework on environmental health economics *(143)*. Finally, a Regional Office publication quantifying the burden of disease from environmental noise *(144)* won an award in the 2012 BMA Medical Book Awards competition.

7. GOVERNANCE, PARTNERSHIPS AND COMMUNICATION

As this report shows, the WHO Regional Office for Europe performed all its work in 2012–2013 with Member States and partners, and as part of one WHO. To increase its effectiveness, it continued to seek sustainable funding, deepen and extend its partnerships, and strengthen its communications. (In April 2013, the Regional Office moved its head office in Copenhagen to the new UN City, housing all the United Nations agencies in Denmark, from the premises it had occupied since 1957, remaining operational throughout the process *(145)*.)

Stronger governance in line with WHO reform

Participating fully in the WHO reform processes *(146)*, the Regional Office pursued three interlocking types of reform (programmatic, governance and managerial), and continued the progress made since the 2010 Regional Committee session in ensuring the full participation of all Member States.

Programmatic reform

To provide input from the European Region to the January 2013 meeting of the WHO Executive

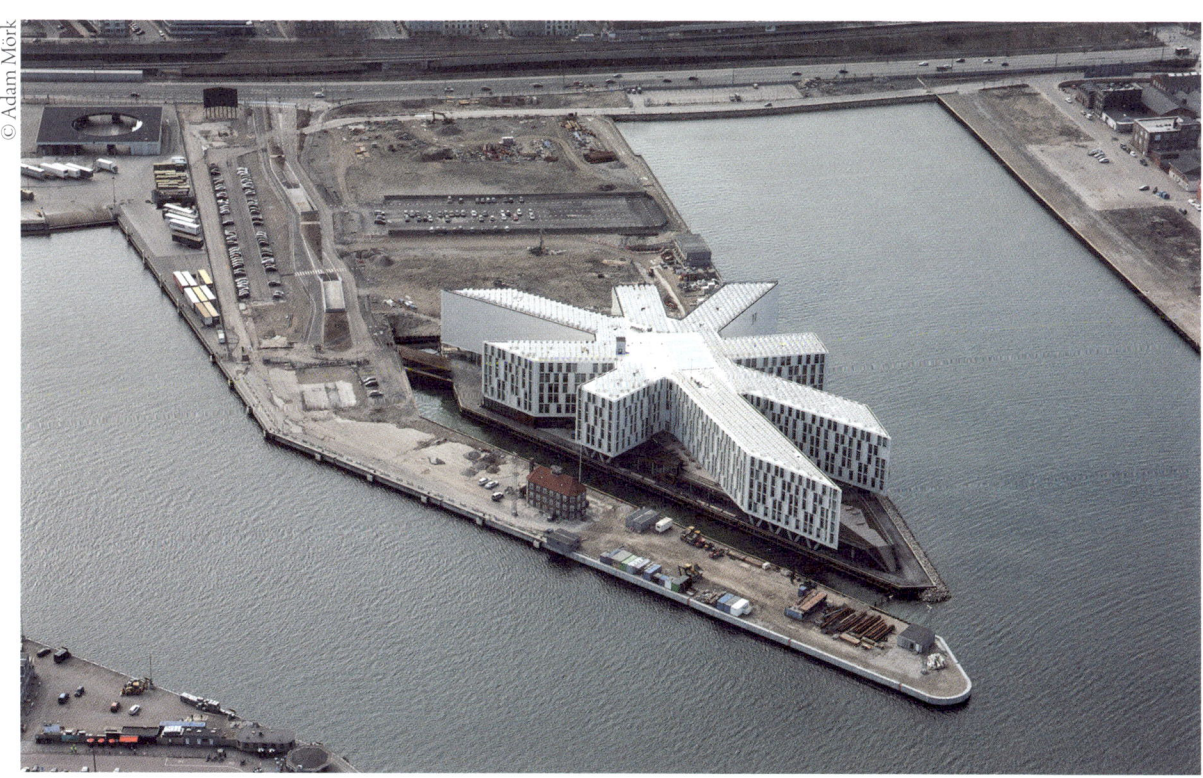

Board and its Programme, Budget and Administration Committee (PBAC), the Regional Office opened a full day of the 2012 Regional Committee session to discussion of:

- the Twelfth General Programme of Work for 2014–2019 (GPW) and the proposed programme budget for 2014–2015 *(147,148)*, and the Regional Office's perspective on the budget *(149)*; and
- measures to improve the predictability, flexibility and sustainability of WHO's financing.

Seizing this opportunity, the Regional Committee welcomed the GPW and budget documents, but asked for further clarification of WHO's strategic direction, detailed information on costs and budget allocation between priorities, greater transparency about the resources available and greater clarity about the division of labour between WHO's three levels *(6)*. In addition, representatives suggested two changes to WHO's current practices to ensure that priority work was properly funded:

- to fill gaps by allocating assessed contributions and funds from the core voluntary contributions account after earmarked voluntary contributions had been determined; and
- to bring the implementation of budgets approved by the World Health Assembly closer to the date of adoption by changing the start of WHO's financial year *(6)*.

Approved by the 2013 World Health Assembly, the GPW comprised WHO's roadmap through to 2019 and the programme budget for 2014–2015 (the first to cover both assessed and voluntary contributions), set out the roles of its global, regional and country offices and laid the foundation for greater transparency, accountability and oversight by governing bodies *(146)*. Building on these, the Regional Office focused on operational planning for 2014–2015 in the second half of 2013, even though the final allocation of resources would not be made until the financing dialogue with donors had been completed at the end of the year *(146,147)*. Two features informed this planning, and reform-related activities as a whole in the European Region:

- the Regional Office's business model, which enabled it to stretch modest resources to serve many countries primarily by addressing their common needs through Region-wide approaches and an intercountry or multicountry mode of programme delivery; and
- its use of Health 2020 as the guiding framework for all policies, strategies and programmes in the Region, fully aligned with global developments.

The Regional Office held a ten-day Office-wide retreat, with the participation of the heads of the Region's 29 country offices, to discuss regional coherence, particularly in implementing Health 2020.

Because the way in which WHO planned its work, obtained its finances and distributed resources internally needed further reform, the Regional Office began work not only to find resources for strategic objectives underfunded for 2014–2015 but also to develop a new bottom-up planning process for preparing the programme budget for 2016–2017, and methodologies for strategic results-based allocation of resources and better management of overhead costs.

The 2013 Regional Committee spent a half-day discussing WHO reform, particularly to review: the impact of WHO reform on the Regional Office; the implementation of the programme budget for 2014–2015 *(150,151)*, including strategic resource allocation, and the Regional Office's financial situation; the process for developing the programme budget for 2016–2017; and the outcome of the first meeting of the financing dialogue (discussed below). The Regional Committee concluded that the reform process was making WHO more effective, transparent, accountable and financially consistent, congratulated both countries and the Secretariat on the progress achieved so far and strongly supported the processes and methodologies under development *(7)*.

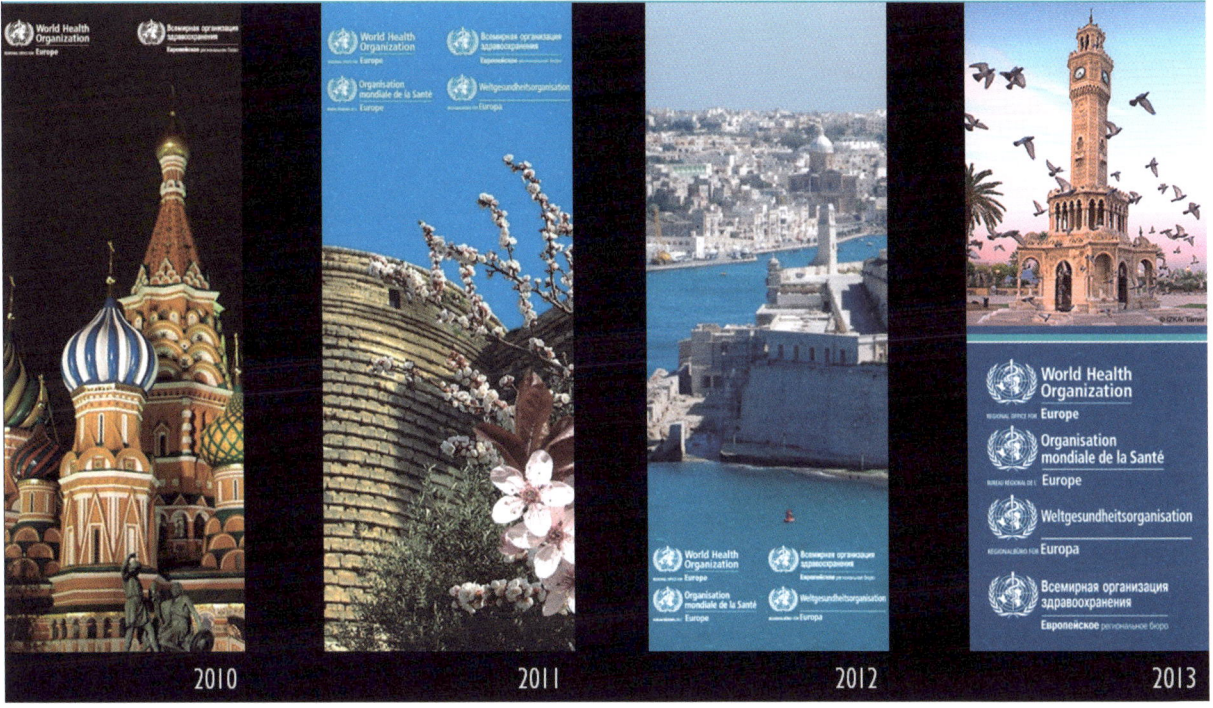

Governance reform

Governance reform comprises both WHO's internal governance and its role on the global health stage. This section addresses the first of these; the second is covered in the section below on partnerships.

With guidance from the Regional Committee and the SCRC, the Regional Office pursued both WHO reform and greater coherence and better governance in its own work. For example, the Regional Director took part in meetings of the Global Policy Group (GPG) and co-chaired the WHO Task Force on Resource Mobilization and Management Strategies, with participation from all regions and major offices. To prepare for the final discussion of the GPW and programme budget by the 2013 World Health Assembly, the Regional Office consulted Member States in April to discuss WHO financing *(10)*.

The Regional Office continued its work to ensure the full participation of all Member States by strengthening the decision-making role of the regional governing bodies, and increasing their transparency, as well as the Secretariat's accountability to them *(1,2)*. In addition to the measures begun in 2010–2011 *(5)*, it supported the SCRC subgroup on governance, which proposed improvements to procedures in seven areas *(152)*:

- the process for nominations to the SCRC and the Executive Board;
- the transparency of SCRC proceedings;
- deadlines for both submission and amendment of Regional Committee resolutions;
- the credentials of Member States attending Regional Committee sessions;
- communication between SCRC members and Member States;
- the code of conduct for nomination of the Regional Director; and
- the staggered replacement of members of the European Environment and Health Ministerial Board (as mentioned in Chapter 6).

In addition, the Regional Office presented a review of the 46 Regional Committee resolutions from the last 10 years that were currently in force, and made recommendations on streamlining requirements for reporting on and setting end dates for these and future resolutions *(153)*. The 2013 Regional Committee approved the SCRC proposals, welcoming the increased transparency and opportunity to be more involved in SCRC discussions, and those made in the review of resolutions *(7)*. In addition, the Regional Office used innovative tools, such as Twitter, Facebook and live webcasts of Regional Committee and ministerial discussions, to add transparency to and enable civil-society organizations and other stakeholders to participate in the governance and decision-making processes.

Managerial reform

The Regional Office played its part in work for managerial reform – to ensure the predictability, transparency and flexibility of the future financing of WHO – in both the European Region and globally. It worked through established channels, such as WHO's governing bodies, and new ones, such as the WHO Task Force on Resource Mobilization and Management Strategies and the 2013 financing dialogue with potential donors. Work in these channels was linked: regional committees' comments on the first financing dialogue in June 2013 provided structured input into the second dialogue in November, and in 2014 the Executive Board and the World Health Assembly would review the lessons learnt.

WHO convened a financing dialogue both with and among Member States and other funders in June and November 2013 *(146,154)*. The participants represented many Member States, other United Nations agencies and non-State partner organizations. At the first meeting, they specifically committed themselves:

- to respect the programmatic priorities set by the World Health Assembly;
- to increase the predictability of their contributions, for example by making public their provisional commitments and moving towards multiyear commitments;
- to increase the flexibility of their funding, for example by raising the level of earmarking;
- to broaden the base of contributors;
- to increase transparency and accountability around WHO financing through such means as a web portal that WHO was developing to provide access to real-time results and programmatic, budgetary and financial and monitoring information; and
- to continue the discussion in WHO regional committees.

WHO agreed to follow up by: launching the web portal *(155)*, starting a bottom-up process for operational planning, conducting bilateral follow-up with Member States and other funders, reporting to regional committees, working to broaden the contributors base and taking a more coordinated approach to resource mobilization and income planning across all levels of the Organization, as well as planning for the work beyond the second meeting in the financing dialogue. The 2013 WHO Regional Committee for Europe welcomed WHO's efforts to mobilize resources, and supported the key commitments made during the financing dialogue, particularly: aligning resources with national priorities, increasing transparency and accountability through the web portal and widening the donor base *(7)*. After the Regional Committee session, the SCRC established a subgroup on allocation of flexible resources to ensure continuous, stable allocation of funding for implementation of the GPW *(10)*.

WHO held the second meeting in the financing dialogue with feedback from its regional committees; 266 participants from 92 Member States and non-State partners attended in person or by webcast *(146)*. Member States and other funders – particularly non-State actors such as the Bill & Melinda Gates Foundation, the GAVI Alliance, Rotary International and UNITAID (a global health initiative) – pledged to provide close to 85% of funding for 2014–2015. Nevertheless, the participants recognized that achieving full alignment of resources was WHO's biggest financing challenge; steps suggested to surmount this included the possible reallocation of resources to underfunded areas. In view of the vulnerability of WHO funding, concluding the framework for engaging with non-State actors was imperative. In addition, the participants supported:

- the move towards an integrated budget;
- the attribution of the costs of programme administration and management to each category of work and their inclusion in agreements on voluntary contributions;
- the framework for a coordinated approach to resource mobilization to fill budget shortfalls, which was presented by the WHO Regional Director for Europe; and
- the Secretariat's vision for improving WHO's reporting and reducing its transaction costs.

WHO pledged to take a variety of steps to follow up the progress made in the financing dialogues, to address budget shortfalls, evaluate the dialogue and continue it with all contributors and inform Member States about the progress made in meetings of WHO governing bodies in 2014.

Reflecting on the dialogue, the Regional Director concluded that the process showed that WHO had built increased trust with donors, and was shifting towards a unified, corporate approach to resource mobilization. This process was not complete, however; pledges had to be converted into contributions, and in 2014 the GPG needed to determine how to distribute resources equitably within WHO, work that included eliminating the pockets of poverty to be found in every office.

Financial overview

During the biennium, the Regional Office's budget as approved by the World Health Assembly – US$ 213 million – was increased by US$ 40 million

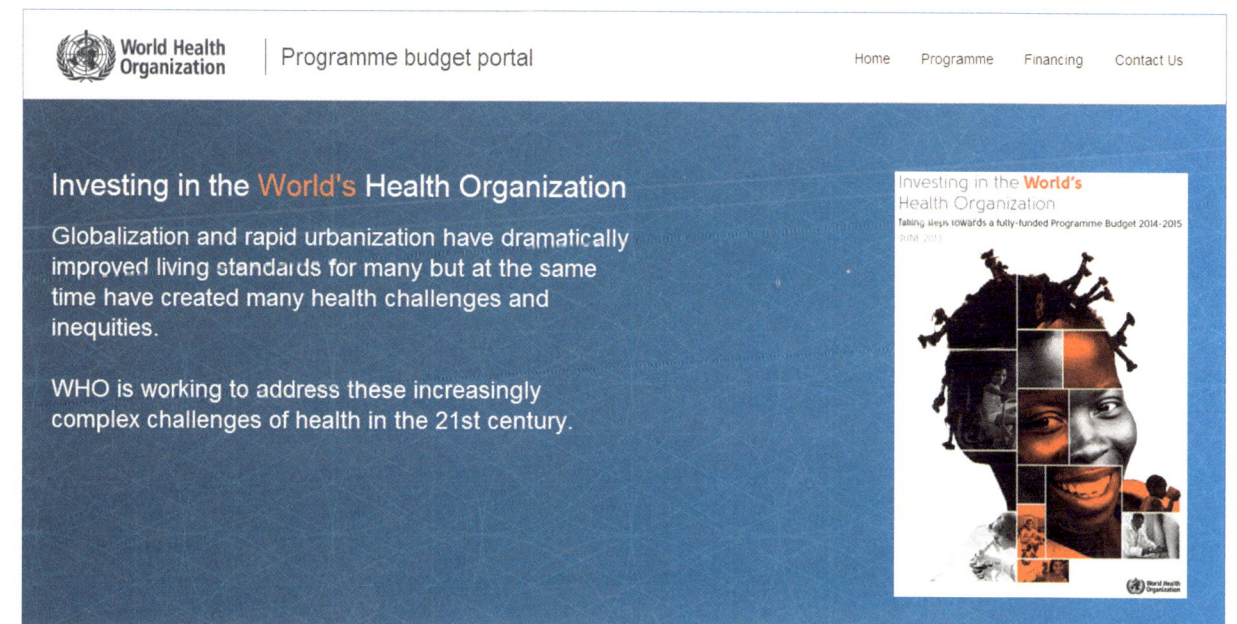

(19%), resulting in an allocated budget of US$ 253 million. The WHO Director-General authorized the budget envelope increases on the basis of a combination of programme and funding opportunities and some large single-country projects.

By 31 December 2013, the Regional Office's budget as approved by the World Health Assembly was funded at 104%, while the current allocated budget of US$ 253 million was funded at 87%. The illustrations in the Annex show the Regional Office's progress in implementing the programme budget for 2012–2013. Overall, 97% of the budget approved by the World Health Assembly was implemented.

Challenges in 2012–2013 included:

- "pockets of poverty": overall funding was good but specific programmes were underfunded;
- earmarking: only 12% of available voluntary contributions to the Regional Office were fully flexible, while the remaining funds were tightly earmarked;
- resource mobilization: as noted, the Director-General set up a task force to address this issue;
- full cost recovery: funding arrangements in some areas did not allow for the covering of salary gaps in specific technical programmes; and
- increased staff costs, despite reductions in staff numbers, due to factors such as exchange rates that are beyond WHO's control.

To improve the situation for 2014–2015, the Regional Office took measures to lower staff costs by reducing recruitment, while trying to preserve technical capacity. In particular, it sought to reduce the costs of administrative staff without overburdening technical staff. The Regional Office developed a new mechanism for donor proposal agreements, which aimed to improve the quality of resources and match them to the priorities approved by Member States. In the short term, it also took measures to save money (by reducing travel costs and spending on consultant services) in ways that would not prejudice the Regional Office's ability to meet its commitments to Member States.

Deepening partnerships

Part of WHO's work in governance reform was to clarify its role on the global health stage: defining its responsibilities among the growing number of organizations working for international health.

This report clearly shows the range, depth and growing specificity of the Regional Office's work with partners such as other United Nations agencies; global health partnerships, particularly the Global Fund, GAVI Alliance and STOP TB partnership; subregional networks such as SEEHN, the Northern Dimension Partnership in Public Health and Social Well-being and the CIS health council and civil-society organizations. In addition to joint activities with, for example, OECD, UNICEF and UNFPA, the Regional Office signed detailed plans for joint action with these organizations at the 2012 and 2013 Regional Committee sessions, as described above *(6,7)*.

In particular, the Regional Office strengthened its cooperation with the EU and its institutions, including the European Parliament. It made major progress in implementing the joint roadmaps agreed with the EC, which facilitate the achievement of the joint declaration signed at the 2010 Regional Committee, and worked closely with ECDC, with which it has joint annual workplans and common guiding principles of collaboration *(5)*. The Regional Office and EFSA agreed to intensify their collaboration, already strong in food safety and antimicrobial resistance related to it, zoonoses and nutrition *(156)*. It continued work with the European Monitoring Centre for Drugs and Drug Addiction (EMCDDA) on health in prisons. In addition, the Regional Office carried out its responsibility for leading relations with the EU and its institutions for all of WHO *(157)*. Finally, the

Governance, partnerships and communication

Regional Office continued support to the health priorities of countries holding the EU Presidency, as described above.

Further, the Regional Office increased its engagement in the United Nations RCM and the regional UNDG. They provide excellent entry points for coordination and are crucial in fostering communication, cooperation and policy coherence. The Regional Office hosted meetings of both in April 2013. Examples of their work include the United Nations interagency working groups on coordinating action towards MDG achievement (under the auspices of the RCM) and on the health of Roma women and children and on tackling inequities (carried out by the regional UNDG's Roma Regional Working Group), discussed in Chapter 1.

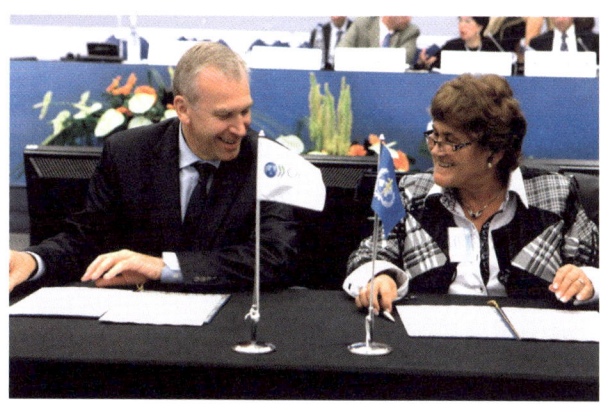

Intensified collaboration with Member States

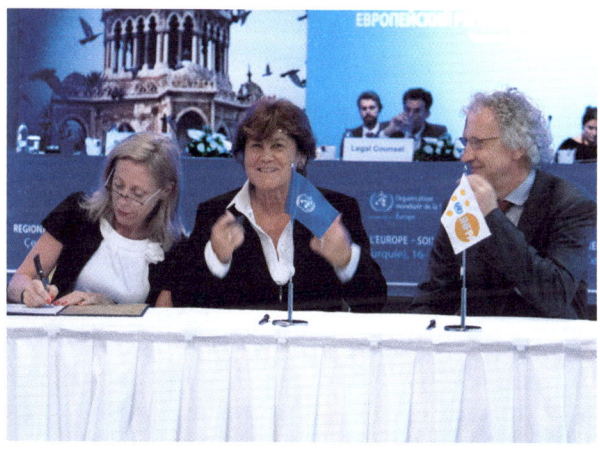

The Regional Office presented an interim strategy on work with countries, drafted with the active participation of Member States and the SCRC and aligned with WHO reform, to the 2012 Regional Committee *(158)*. It set out a number of ways in which the Regional Office could ensure a regular and flexible approach for work for, with and in all 53 countries, including suggestions on working with countries that lack country offices and the tools and instruments that can be used to facilitate this, such as country cooperation strategies (CCSs). The Regional Committee agreed on the value of the CCS as a flexible tool for cooperation between WHO and interested Member States and called for the presentation of a final strategy on work with countries in 2014 *(6)*. In the mean time, the Regional Office started developing CCSs, signing the first with Switzerland in May 2013 *(159)* and beginning to develop others with Belgium, Cyprus, Portugal, the Russian Federation and Turkey.

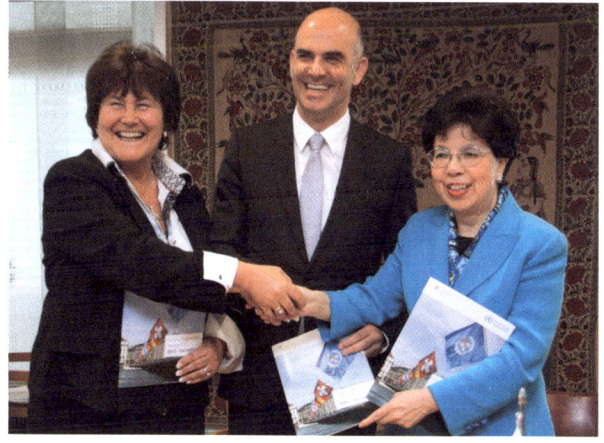

Seeking to address the needs of all 53 Member States, the Regional Office also reinforced the structure of its country presence to provide greater support through provision of training on Health 2020, NCDs and health information. It also continued to implement the biennial collaborative agreements made with over half the countries in the Region and welcomed ministers from a large number of countries on over 30 official visits. In addition, the WHO Regional Director for Europe made over 50 visits to countries and regional or international events.

Strategic communications

In 2012–2013, the Regional Office widened the reach of its messages and deepened engagement with Member States, donors, partners and other stakeholders by conducting its communications strategically and employing innovative communication methods. The Regional Office website *(9)* was the key tool for communicating the work of the entire Office, including its technical divisions and country offices, in support of Member States. The website attracted 18% more traffic in the first 7 months of 2013 than in the same period in 2012, especially during key events. In addition, the Regional Office made its information accessible by mobile devices, and an increased number of stakeholders, surveyed in 2013, were satisfied with the quality, value and accessibility of the information provided.

Publishing remained the primary means through which the WHO Regional Office for Europe spread its messages to and beyond the European Region, and its website was the primary platform for this work *(9,160)*. Regional Office publications were viewed or downloaded more than 300 000 times per year, and two won prizes in the BMA Medical Book Awards competition *(98,144)*. Up to 10 times as many readers accessed the most popular publications online as in printed copies, and the website was essential to the sharing of data and evidence through, for example, the Regional Office's most popular data source, the European Health for All Database *(161)*.

The Regional Office continued showcasing the work done with Member States and other partners, building on its networks and reaching broader audiences by using new, innovative communication methods, including social media such as Facebook and Twitter, along with traditional information and events for the mass media *(162)*. Thanks to months of proactive media work and use of social media, key events such as the launches of the Health 2020 policy framework and the European health report, ministerial conferences, World Health Day and European Immunization Week *(8,11,48,87,101,119)* achieved wide visibility. In addition, the Regional Office's communication and partner networks helped to spread the messages further. During public health emergencies, such as the MERS-CoV outbreak, the Regional Office coordinated communications to Member States and provided reliable, clear information to the mass media and wider audiences, as well as deploying expert staff upon countries' request.

In addition, to facilitate its work and promote a positive working environment, the Regional Office began developing a comprehensive internal communications strategy, optimizing the use of the intranet as a key platform and increasing information sharing and interaction between all WHO offices in the Region.

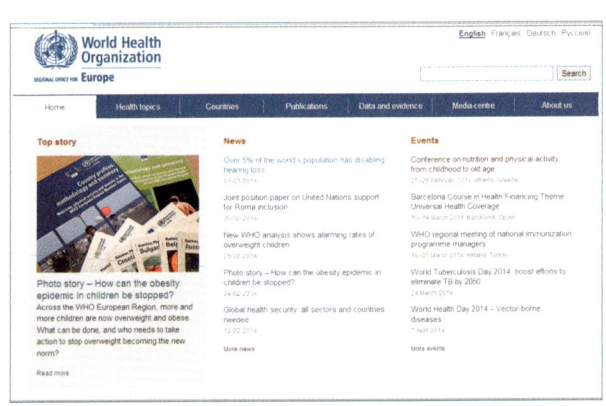

REFERENCES[1]

1. Better health for Europe: adapting the Regional Office for Europe to the changing European environment: the Regional Director's perspective. Copenhagen: WHO Regional Office for Europe; 2010 (EUR/RC60/8; http://www.euro.who.int/en/who-we-are/governance/regional-committee-for-europe/past-sessions/sixtieth-session/documentation/working-documents/eurrc608).

2. Report of the sixtieth session of the WHO Regional Committee for Europe. Copenhagen: WHO Regional Office for Europe; 2010 (http://www.euro.who.int/en/who-we-are/governance/regional-committee-for-europe/past-sessions/sixtieth-session/documentation/report-of-the-sixtieth-session2).

3. The first six months. Copenhagen: WHO Regional Office for Europe; 2010 (http://www.euro.who.int/__data/assets/pdf_file/0003/122907/who-RD-brochure-UK-www.pdf).

4. Report of the sixty-first session of the WHO Regional Committee for Europe. Copenhagen: WHO Regional Office for Europe; 2011 (http://www.euro.who.int/en/who-we-are/governance/regional-committee-for-europe/sixty first-session/documentation/report-of-the-sixty-first-session-of-the-who-regional-committee-for-europe).

5. What we've achieved together: report of the Regional Director on the work of WHO in the European Region in 2010–2011. Copenhagen: WHO Regional Office for Europe; 2012 (http://www.euro.who.int/en/what-we-publish/abstracts/what-weve-achieved-together-report-of-the-regional-director-on-the-work-of-who-in-the-european-region-in-20102011).

6. Report of the sixty-second session of the WHO Regional Committee for Europe. Copenhagen: WHO Regional Office for Europe; 2012 (http://www.euro.who.int/en/about-us/governance/regional-committee-for-europe/sixty-second-session/documentation/report-of-the-sixty-second-session-of-the-who-regional-committee-for-europe).

7. Report of the sixty-third session of the WHO Regional Committee for Europe. Copenhagen: WHO Regional Office for Europe; 2013 (http://www.euro.who.int/en/about-us/governance/regional-committee-for-europe/sixty-third-session/report-of-the-sixty-third-session-of-the-who-regional-committee-for-europe).

8. The European health report 2012: charting the way to well-being. Copenhagen: WHO Regional Office for Europe; 2013 (http://www.euro.who.int/en/data-and-evidence/european-health-report-2012).

9. WHO Regional Office for Europe [website]. Copenhagen: WHO Regional Office for Europe; 2013 (http://www.euro.who.int/en/home).

10. Standing Committee [website]. Copenhagen: WHO Regional Office for Europe; 2013 (http://www.euro.who.int/en/about-us/governance/standing-committee).

1 All electronic references were accessed on 19 March 2014.

11. Health 2020. A European policy framework and strategy for the 21st century. Copenhagen: WHO Regional Office for Europe; 2013 (http://www.euro.who.int/en/health-topics/health-policy/health-2020-the-european-policy-for-health-and-well-being/publications/2013/health-2020-a-european-policy-framework-and-strategy-for-the-21st-century).

12. Executive summary of the European health report 2012: moving Europe towards health and well-being. Copenhagen: WHO Regional Office for Europe; 2012 (EUR/RC62/Inf.Doc./1; http://www.euro.who.int/en/who-we-are/governance/regional-committee-for-europe/sixty-second-session/documentation/information-documents/eurrc62inf.doc.1-executive-summary-of-the-european-health-report-2012-moving-europe-towards-health-and-well-being).

13. The evidence base of Health 2020. Copenhagen: WHO Regional Office for Europe; 2012 (EUR/RC62/Inf.Doc./2; http://www.euro.who.int/en/who-we-are/governance/regional-committee-for-europe/sixty-second-session/documentation/information-documents/eurrc62inf.doc.2-the-evidence-base-of-health-2020).

14. Implementing Health 2020. Copenhagen: WHO Regional Office for Europe; 2012 (EUR/RC62/Inf.Doc./3; http://www.euro.who.int/en/who-we-are/governance/regional-committee-for-europe/sixty-second-session/documentation/information-documents/eurrc62inf.doc.3-implementing-health-2020).

15. Monitoring framework for Health 2020 targets and indicators. Copenhagen: WHO Regional Office for Europe; 2012 (EUR/RC62/Inf.Doc./4; http://www.euro.who.int/en/who-we-are/governance/regional-committee-for-europe/sixty-second-session/documentation/information-documents/eurrc62inf.doc.4-monitoring-framework-for-health-2020-targets-and-indicators).

16. The Tallinn Charter: Health Systems for Health and Wealth. Copenhagen: WHO Regional Office for Europe; 2008 (http://www.euro.who.int/en/who-we-are/policy-documents/tallinn-charter-health-systems-for-health-and-wealth).

17. European Action Plan for Strengthening Public Health Capacities and Services. Copenhagen: WHO Regional Office for Europe; 2012 (http://www.euro.who.int/en/what-we-do/health-topics/Health-systems/public-health-services/publications2/2012/european-action-plan-for-strengthening-public-health-capacities-and-services).

18. WHO Regional Committee for Europe resolution EUR/RC62/R4 on Health 2020 – The European policy framework for health and well-being. Copenhagen: WHO Regional Office for Europe; 2012 (http://www.euro.who.int/en/who-we-are/governance/regional-committee-for-europe/sixty-second-session/documentation/resolutions-and-decisions/eurrc62r4-health-2020-the-european-policy-framework-for-health-and-well-being).

19. Review of social determinants and the health divide in the WHO European Region. Final report. Copenhagen: WHO Regional Office for Europe; 2012 (http://www.euro.who.int/en/publications/abstracts/review-of-social-determinants-and-the-health-divide-in-the-who-european-region.-final-report).

20. Report on social determinants of health and the health divide in the WHO European Region. Executive summary. Copenhagen: WHO Regional Office for Europe; 2012 (http://www.euro.who.int/en/who-we-are/governance/regional-committee-for-europe/sixty-second-session/documentation/background-documents/report-on-social-

determinants-of-health-and-the-health-divide-in-the-who-european-region.-executive-summary).

21. Kickbusch I, Gleicher D. Governance for health in the 21st century. Copenhagen: WHO Regional Office for Europe; 2012 (http://www.euro.who.int/en/what-we-publish/abstracts/governance-for-health-in-the-21st-century).

22. Kickbusch I, Behrendt T. Implementing a Health 2020 vision: governance for health in the 21st century. Making it happen. Copenhagen: WHO Regional Office for Europe; 2012 (http://www.euro.who.int/en/publications/abstracts/implementing-a-health-2020-vision-governance-for-health-in-the-21st-century.-making-it-happen).

23. McQueen D, Wismar M, Lin V, Jones CM, Davies M, editors. Intersectoral governance for Health in All Policies. Structures, actions and experiences. Copenhagen: WHO Regional Office for Europe, on behalf of the European Observatory on Health Systems and Policies; 2012 (Observatory Studies Series, No.26; http://www.euro.who.int/en/what-we-publish/abstracts/intersectoral-governance-for-health-in-all-policies.-structures,-actions-and-experiences).

24. McDaid D, Sassi F, Merkur S, editors. Promoting health, preventing disease: the economic case. Maidenhead, Open University Press (in press).

25. Bertollini R, Brassart C, Galanaki C. Review of the commitments of Member States and the WHO Regional Office for Europe between 1990 and 2010: analysis in the light of the Health 2020 strategy. Copenhagen: WHO Regional Office for Europe; 2012 (http://www.euro.who.int/en/who-we-are/governance/regional-committee-for-europe/sixty-second-session/documentation/background-documents/review-of-the-commitments-of-who-european-member-states-and-the-who-regional-office-for-europe-between-1990-and-2010).

26. Health 2020: the European policy for health and well-being [website]. Copenhagen: WHO Regional Office for Europe; 2013 (http://www.euro.who.int/health2020).

27. Implementing Health 2020. Copenhagen: WHO Regional Office for Europe; 2013 (EUR/RC63/Inf.Doc./1; http://www.euro.who.int/en/about-us/governance/regional-committee-for-europe/sixty-third-session/documentation/information-documents/eurrc63inf.doc.1-implementing-health-2020).

28. Developing countries' capacity to implement Health 2020 [website]. Copenhagen: WHO Regional Office for Europe; 2013 (http://www.euro.who.int/en/health-topics/health-policy/health-2020-the-european-policy-for-health-and-well-being/news/news/2014/01/developing-countries-capacity-to-implement-health-2020).

29. Report. Third meeting of the European Health Policy Forum of High-Level Government Officials. Copenhagen: WHO Regional Office for Europe; 2012 (http://www.euro.who.int/en/who-we-are/governance/regional-committee-for-europe/news/news/2012/4/forum-finalizes-health-2020-policy-framework/report-third-meeting-of-the-european-health-policy-forum-of-high-level-government-officials).

30. Measurement of and target-setting for well-being: an initiative by the WHO Regional Office for Europe. First meeting of the expert group, Copenhagen, Denmark, 8–9 February 2012. Copenhagen: WHO Regional Office for Europe; 2012 (http://www.euro.who.int/en/health-topics/health-determinants/social-determinants/activities/data-analysis-and-monitoring/measurement-of-and-target-setting-for-well-being-an-initiative-by-the-who-regional-office-for-europe/first-meeting-of-the-expert-group,-copenhagen,-denmark,-89-february-2012).

31. Measurement of and target-setting for well-being: an initiative by the WHO Regional Office for Europe. Second meeting of the expert group, Paris, France, 25–26 June 2012. Copenhagen: WHO Regional Office for Europe; 2013 (http://www.euro.who.int/en/publications/abstracts/measurement-of-and-target-setting-for-well-being-an-initiative-by-the-who-regional-office-for-europe).

32. Joint meeting of experts on targets and indicators for health and well-being in Health 2020. Copenhagen: WHO Regional Office for Europe; 2013 (http://www.euro.who.int/en/what-we-publish/abstracts/joint-meeting-of-experts-on-targets-and-indicators-for-health-and-well-being-in-health-2020).

33. NCD Global Monitoring Framework. Ensuring progress on noncommunicable diseases in countries [website]. Geneva: World Health Organization; 2013 (http://www.who.int/nmh/global_monitoring_framework/en).

34. Core health indicators in the WHO European Region 2013. Special focus: noncommunicable diseases. Copenhagen: WHO Regional Office for Europe; 2013 (http://www.euro.who.int/en/data-and-evidence/core-health-indicators-in-the-who-european-region-2013.-special-focus-noncommunicable-diseases).

35. WHO Regional Committee for Europe resolution EUR/RC63/R3 on indicators for Health 2020 targets. Copenhagen: WHO Regional Office for Europe; 2013 (http://www.euro.who.int/en/about-us/governance/regional-committee-for-europe/sixty-third-session/documentation/resolutions-and-decisions/eurrc63r3-indicators-for-health-2020-targets).

36. Vulnerability and health: WHO opens new collaborating centre in Hungary [website]. Copenhagen: WHO Regional Office for Europe; 2012 (http://www.euro.who.int/en/what-we-do/health-topics/health-determinants/social-determinants/news/news/2012/02/vulnerability-and-health-who-opens-new-collaborating-centre-in-hungary).

37. Migration and health [website]. Copenhagen: WHO Regional Office for Europe; 2013 (http://www.euro.who.int/en/health-topics/health-determinants/migration-and-health).

38. Human Rights Day 2012: "My voice counts" [website]. Copenhagen: WHO Regional Office for Europe; 2012 (http://www.euro.who.int/en/what-we-do/health-topics/health-determinants/social-determinants/news/news/2012/12/human-rights-day-2012-my-voice-counts).

39. Roma health newsletter [website]. Copenhagen: WHO Regional Office for Europe; 2012 (http://www.euro.who.int/en/what-we-publish/newsletters/roma-health-newsletter).

40. Roma health mediation in Romania. Copenhagen: WHO Regional Office for Europe; 2013 (Roma Health – Case Study Series No. 1; http://www.euro.who.int/en/publications/abstracts/roma-health-mediation-in-romania).

41. Progress towards Millennium Development Goals 4, 5 and 6 in the WHO European Region: 2011 update. Copenhagen: WHO Regional Office for Europe; 2012 (http://www.euro.who.int/en/what-we-do/health-topics/health-determinants/millenium-development-goals/publications2/2012/progress-towards-millennium-development-goals-4,-5-and-6-in-the-who-european-region-2011-update).

42. Significant progress in implementing activities for Roma health [website]. Copenhagen: WHO Regional Office for Europe; 2013 (http://

References

www.euro.who.int/en/about-us/partners/news/news/2013/07/significant-progress-in-implementing-activities-for-roma-health).

43. Review of public health capacities and services in the European Region. Copenhagen: WHO Regional Office for Europe; 2012 (http://www.euro.who.int/en/what-we-do/health-topics/Health-systems/public-health-services/publications2/2012/review-of-public-health-capacities-and-services-in-the-european-region).

44. Preliminary review of institutional models for delivering essential public health operations in Europe. Copenhagen: WHO Regional Office for Europe; 2012 (http://www.euro.who.int/en/what-we-do/health-topics/Health-systems/public-health-services/publications2/2012/preliminary-review-of-institutional-models-for-delivering-essential-public-health-operations-in-europe).

45. Public health policy and legislation instruments and tools: an updated review and proposal for further research. Copenhagen: WHO Regional Office for Europe; 2012 (http://www.euro.who.int/en/what-we-do/health-topics/Health-systems/public-health-services/publications2/2012/public-health-policy-and-legislation-instruments-and-tools-an-updated-review-and-proposal-for-further-research).

46. Public health services [website]. Copenhagen: WHO Regional Office for Europe; 2013 (http://www.euro.who.int/public-health-services).

47. Health systems financing [website]. Copenhagen: WHO Regional Office for Europe; 2013 (http://www.euro.who.int/en/what-we-do/health-topics/Health-systems/health-systems-financing).

48. Strengthening people-centred health systems in the WHO European Region: a roadmap. Copenhagen: WHO Regional Office for Europe; 2013 (http://www.euro.who.int/en/media-centre/events/events/2013/10/health-systems-for-health-and-wealth-in-the-context-of-health-2020/documentation/background-documents/strengthening-people-centred-health-systems-in-the-who-european-region-a-roadmap).

49. Make health systems people centred [website]. Copenhagen: WHO Regional Office for Europe; 2013 (http://www.euro.who.int/en/health-topics/Health-systems/health-systems-governance/news/news/2013/10/make-health-systems-people-centred).

50. Declaration of Alma-Ata, 1978. Copenhagen: WHO Regional Office for Europe; 2013 (http://www.euro.who.int/en/publications/policy-documents/declaration-of-alma-ata,-1978).

51. Greece [website]. Copenhagen: WHO Regional Office for Europe; 2013 (http://www.euro.who.int/en/countries/greece).

52. A review of health financing reforms in the Republic of Moldova. Copenhagen: WHO Regional Office for Europe; 2012 (Health Financing Policy Paper 2012/1; http://www.euro.who.int/en/what-we-do/health-topics/Health-systems/health-systems-financing/publications2/2012/20121-a-review-of-health-financing-reforms-in-the-republic-of-moldova).

53. Behind the estimates of out-of-pocket spending on health in the former Soviet Union. Copenhagen: WHO Regional Office for Europe; 2012 (Health Financing Policy Paper 2011/1; http://www.euro.who.int/en/what-we-do/health-topics/Health-systems/health-systems-financing/publications2/2012/20111-behind-the-estimates-of-out-of-pocket-spending-on-health-in-the-former-soviet-union).

54. Impact of the financial crisis on health and health systems [website]. Copenhagen: WHO Regional Office for Europe; 2013 (http://www.euro.who.int/en/what-we-do/health-topics/Health-systems/health-systems-financing/activities/impact-of-the-financial-crisis-on-health-and-health-systems).

55. Thomson S, Jowett M, Mladovsky P, editors. Health system responses to financial pressures in Ireland: policy options in an international context. Copenhagen: WHO Regional Office for Europe; 2012 (http://www.dohc.ie/publications/pdf/Observatory_WHO_2012.pdf?direct=1).

56. Health, health systems and economic crisis in Europe: impact and policy implications. Copenhagen: WHO Regional Office for Europe; 2013 (http://www.euro.who.int/en/media-centre/events/events/2013/04/oslo-conference-on-health-systems-and-the-economic-crisis/documentation/working-documents/health,-health-systems-and-economic-crisis-in-europe-impact-and-policy-implications).

57. Health systems in times of global economic crisis: an update of the situation in the WHO European Region [website]. Copenhagen: WHO Regional Office for Europe; 2013 (http://www.euro.who.int/en/what-we-do/event/oslo-conference-on-health-systems-and-the-economic-crisis).

58. Reigniting economic growth and reducing unemployment are good health policy [website]. Copenhagen: WHO Regional Office for Europe; 2013 (http://www.euro.who.int/en/what-we-do/health-topics/Health-systems/health-systems-financing/news/news/2013/04/reigniting-economic-growth-and-reducing-unemployment-are-good-health-policy).

59. Outcome document for the high-level meeting on Health systems in times of global economic crisis: an update of the situation in the WHO European Region. Copenhagen: WHO Regional Office for Europe; 2013 (EUR/RC63/13; http://www.euro.who.int/en/who-we-are/governance/regional-committee-for-europe/sixty-third-session/working-documents/eurrc6313-outcome-document-for-the-high-level-meeting-on-health-systems-in-times-of-global-economic-crisis-an-update-of-the-situation-in-the-who-european-region).

60. Barcelona Course on Health Financing [website]. Copenhagen: WHO Regional Office for Europe; 2013 (http://www.euro.who.int/en/health-topics/Health-systems/health-systems-financing/activities/learning-opportunities-and-training-courses/barcelona-course-on-health-financing).

61. Flagship Course on Health System Strengthening [website]. Copenhagen: WHO Regional Office for Europe; 2013 (http://www.euro.who.int/en/health-topics/Health-systems/health-systems-financing/activities/learning-opportunities-and-training-courses/flagship-course-on-health-system-strengthening).

62. Health workforce [website]. Copenhagen: WHO Regional Office for Europe; 2013 (http://www.euro.who.int/en/what-we-do/health-topics/Health-systems/health-workforce).

63. WHO policy dialogue on international health workforce mobility and recruitment challenges technical report. Copenhagen: WHO Regional Office for Europe; 2013 (http://www.euro.who.int/en/health-topics/Health-systems/health-workforce/publications2/2013/who-policy-dialogue-on-international-health-workforce-mobility-and-recruitment-challenges-technical-report).

64. SOM 2012: Update on the Roadmap for EC/WHO/Europe collaboration on modernizing and integrating the public health information system

References

[website]. Copenhagen: WHO Regional Office for Europe; 2013 (http://www.euro.who.int/en/who-we-are/partners/other-partners/european-union-eu-and-its-institutions2/european-commission-ec/senior-officials-meeting-som-2012/update-on-the-roadmaps-for-ec-whoeurope-collaboration/som-2012-update-on-the-roadmap-for-ecwhoeurope-collaboration-on-modernizing-and-integrating-the-public-health-information-system).

65. Data and evidence [website]. Copenhagen: WHO Regional Office for Europe; 2013 (http://www.euro.who.int/en/what-we-do/data-and-evidence).

66. European database on human and technical resources for health (HlthRes-DB) [online database]. Copenhagen: WHO Regional Office for Europe; 2013 (http://www.euro.who.int/en/data-and-evidence/databases/european-database-on-human-and-technical-resources-for-health-hlthres-db).

67. EVIPNet: putting evidence into policy [website]. Copenhagen: WHO Regional Office for Europe; 2012 (http://www.euro.who.int/en/what-we-do/data-and-evidence/health-evidence-network-hen/sections/news/2012/10/evipnet-putting-evidence-into-policy).

68. Translating evidence into effective public health policy [website]. Copenhagen: WHO Regional Office for Europe; 2013 (http://www.euro.who.int/en/media-centre/sections/press-releases/2013/10/translating-evidence-into-effective-public-health-policy).

69. Action Plan for implementation of the European Strategy for the Prevention and Control of Noncommunicable Diseases 2012–2016. Copenhagen: WHO Regional Office for Europe; 2012 (http://www.euro.who.int/en/what-we-publish/abstracts/action-plan-for-implementation-of-the-european-strategy-for-the-prevention-and-control-of-noncommunicable-diseases-20122016).

70. Political Declaration of the High-level Meeting of the General Assembly on the Prevention and Control of Non-communicable Diseases. New York: United Nations; 2011 (document A/66/L.1; http://www.un.org/ga/search/view_doc.asp?symbol=A/66/L.1).

71. Web consultation on the global monitoring framework for noncommunicable diseases. Copenhagen: WHO Regional Office for Europe; 2012 (http://www.euro.who.int/en/what-we-do/health-topics/noncommunicable-diseases/resolutions-and-meeting-reports/web-consultation-on-the-global-monitoring-framework-for-noncommunicable-diseases).

72. Noncommunicable diseases prevention and control in the South-eastern Europe Health Network. An analysis of intersectoral collaboration. Copenhagen: WHO Regional Office for Europe; 2012 (http://www.euro.who.int/en/what-we-publish/abstracts/noncommunicable-diseases-prevention-and-control-in-the-south-eastern-europe-health-network.-an-analysis-of-intersectoral-collaboration).

73. WHO European Ministerial Conference on the Prevention and Control of Noncommunicable Diseases in the Context of Health 2020 [website]. Copenhagen: WHO Regional Office for Europe; 2013 (http://www.euro.who.int/en/media-centre/events/events/2013/12/ashgabat-conference-on-noncommunicable-diseases).

74. European tobacco control status report 2013. Copenhagen: WHO Regional Office for Europe; 2013 (http://www.euro.who.int/en/health-topics/disease-prevention/tobacco/publications/2013/who-european-tobacco-control-status-report-2013).

75. Ashgabat Declaration on the Prevention and Control of Noncommunicable Diseases in the Context of Health 2020. Copenhagen: WHO Regional Office for Europe; 2013 (http://www.euro.who.int/en/publications/policy-documents/ashgabat-declaration-on-the-prevention-and-control-of-noncommunicable-diseases-in-the-context-of-health-2020).

76. European action plan to reduce the harmful use of alcohol 2012–2020. Copenhagen: WHO Regional Office for Europe; 2012 (http://www.euro.who.int/en/what-we-do/health-topics/disease-prevention/alcohol-use/publications/2012/european-action-plan-to-reduce-the-harmful-use-of-alcohol-20122021).

77. Anderson P, Møller L, Galea G, editors. Alcohol in the European Union. Consumption, harm and policy approaches. Copenhagen: WHO Regional Office for Europe; 2012 (http://www.euro.who.int/en/what-we-publish/abstracts/alcohol-in-the-european-union.-consumption,-harm-and-policy-approaches).

78. Alcohol problems in the criminal justice system: an opportunity for intervention. Copenhagen: WHO Regional Office for Europe; 2013 (http://www.euro.who.int/en/what-we-do/health-topics/disease-prevention/alcohol-use/publications/2013/alcohol-problems-in-the-criminal-justice-system-an-opportunity-for-intervention).

79. WHO Meeting of the National Counterparts for Alcohol Policy in the WHO European Region. Copenhagen: WHO Regional Office for Europe; 2012 (http://www.euro.who.int/en/what-we-do/health-topics/disease-prevention/alcohol-use/publications/2012/who-meeting-of-the-national-counterparts-for-alcohol-policy-in-the-who-european-region).

80. WHO network meeting of National Focal Points for Alcohol Policy and Global Alcohol Policy Symposium, 25–27 April 2013, Istanbul, Turkey. Copenhagen: WHO Regional Office for Europe; 2013 (http://www.euro.who.int/en/what-we-do/health-topics/disease-prevention/alcohol-use/news/news/2013/04/who-network-meeting-of-national-focal-points-for-alcohol-policy-and-global-alcohol-policy-symposium-25-27-april-2013,-istanbul,-turkey).

81. Status report on alcohol and health in 35 European countries 2013. Copenhagen: WHO Regional Office for Europe; 2013 (http://www.euro.who.int/en/health-topics/disease-prevention/alcohol-use/publications/2013/status-report-on-alcohol-and-health-in-35-european-countries-2013).

82. WHO Framework Convention on Tobacco Control [website]. Geneva: World Health Organization; 2013 (http://www.who.int/fctc/en).

83. Tobacco control database for the WHO European Region [online database]. Copenhagen: WHO Regional Office for Europe; 2013 (http://data.euro.who.int/tobacco).

84. World No Tobacco Day [website]. Copenhagen: WHO Regional Office for Europe; 2013 (http://www.euro.who.int/en/what-we-do/health-topics/disease-prevention/tobacco/world-no-tobacco-day).

85. European Charter on Counteracting Obesity. Copenhagen: WHO Regional Office for Europe; 2006 (http://www.euro.who.int/en/who-we-are/policy-documents/european-charter-on-counteracting-obesity).

86. WHO European Action Plan for Food and Nutrition Policy 2007–2012. Copenhagen: WHO Regional Office for Europe; 2008 (http://www.euro.who.int/en/what-we-do/health-topics/noncommunicable-diseases/obesity/

publications/pre-2009/who-european-action-plan-for-food-and-nutrition-policy-2007-2012).

87. Vienna conference on nutrition and noncommunicable diseases [website]. Copenhagen: WHO Regional Office for Europe; 2013 (http://www.euro.who.int/en/what-we-do/event/vienna-conference-on-nutrition-and-noncommunicable-diseases).

88. Vienna Declaration on Nutrition and Noncommunicable Diseases in the Context of Health 2020. Copenhagen: WHO Regional Office for Europe; 2013 (http://www.euro.who.int/en/publications/policy-documents/vienna-declaration-on-nutrition-and-noncommunicable-diseases-in-the-context-of-health-2020).

89. World Health Day [website]. Copenhagen: WHO Regional Office for Europe; 2013 (http://www.euro.who.int/en/about-us/whd).

90. Physical activity promotion in socially disadvantaged groups: principles for action. Policy summary. Copenhagen: WHO Regional Office for Europe; 2013 (http://www.euro.who.int/en/health-topics/disease-prevention/physical-activity/publications/2013/physical-activity-promotion-in-socially-disadvantaged-groups-principles-for-action.-policy-summary).

91. Young and physically active: a blueprint for making physical activity appealing to youth. Copenhagen: WHO Regional Office for Europe; 2013 (http://www.euro.who.int/en/health-topics/Life-stages/child-and-adolescent-health/publications/2012/young-and-physically-active-a-blueprint-for-making-physical-activity-appealing-to-youth).

92. The European Mental Health Action Plan. Copenhagen: WHO Regional Office for Europe; 2013 (EUR/RC63/11; http://www.euro.who.int/en/about-us/governance/regional-committee-for-europe/archive/advance-copies-of-documents/eurrc6311-the-european-mental-health-action-plan).

93. Mitis F, Sethi D. European facts and "Global status report on road safety 2013". Copenhagen: WHO Regional Office for Europe; 2013 (http://www.euro.who.int/en/what-we-publish/abstracts/european-facts-and-global-status-report-on-road-safety-2013).

94. European report on preventing child maltreatment. Copenhagen: WHO Regional Office for Europe; 2013 (http://www.euro.who.int/en/publications/abstracts/european-report-on-preventing-child-maltreatment).

95. Child marriage – a threat to health [website]. Copenhagen: WHO Regional Office for Europe; 2013 (http://www.euro.who.int/en/what-we-do/health-topics/Life-stages/sexual-and-reproductive-health/news/news/2012/12/child-marriage-a-threat-to-health).

96. Child marriage. Entre Nous 2012;76 (http://www.euro.who.int/en/what-we-do/health-topics/Life-stages/sexual-and-reproductive-health/publications/entre-nous/entre-nous/child-marriage.-entre-nous-no.-76,-2012).

97. First step to stronger collaboration with UNFPA [website]. Copenhagen: WHO Regional Office for Europe; 2013 (http://www.euro.who.int/en/what-we-do/health-topics/Life-stages/sexual-and-reproductive-health/news/news/2012/12/first-step-to-stronger-collaboration-with-unfpa).

98. Health Behaviour in School-aged Children (HBSC) [website]. Copenhagen: WHO Regional Office for Europe; 2012 (http://www.euro.who.int/en/health-topics/Life-stages/child-and-adolescent-health/adolescent-health/health-behaviour-in-school-aged-children-hbsc2.-who-collaborative-cross-national-study-of-children-aged-1115).

99. Currie C, Zanotti C, Morgan A, Currie D, de Looze M, Roberts C, et al., editors. Social determinants of health and well-being among young people. Health Behaviour in School-aged Children (HBSC) study: international report from the 2009/2010 survey. Copenhagen: WHO Regional Office for Europe; 2012 (http://www.euro.who.int/en/what-we-do/health-topics/Life-stages/child-and-adolescent-health/publications/2012/social-determinants-of-health-and-well-being-among-young-people.-health-behaviour-in-school-aged-children-hbsc-study).

100. Strategy and action plan for healthy ageing in Europe, 2012–2020. Copenhagen: WHO Regional Office for Europe; 2012 (EUR/RC62/10 Rev.1; http://www.euro.who.int/en/who-we-are/governance/regional-committee-for-europe/sixty-second-session/documentation/working-documents/eurrc6210-rev.1-strategy-and-action-plan-for-healthy-ageing-in-europe,-20122020).

101. Regional World Health Day launch: empower older people to participate in policy-making [website]. Copenhagen: WHO Regional Office for Europe; 2013 (http://www.euro.who.int/en/what-we-do/health-topics/Life-stages/healthy-ageing/news/news/2012/04/regional-world-health-day-launch-empower-older-people-to-participate-in-policy-making).

102. Roadmap to prevent and combat drug-resistant tuberculosis. The Consolidated Action Plan to Prevent and Combat Multidrug- and Extensively Drug-Resistant Tuberculosis in the WHO European Region 2011–2015. Copenhagen: WHO Regional Office for Europe; 2011 (http://www.euro.who.int/en/publications/abstracts/roadmap-to-prevent-and-combat-drug-resistant-tuberculosis).

103. European Action Plan for HIV/AIDS 2012–2015. Copenhagen: WHO Regional Office for Europe; 2011 (http://www.euro.who.int/en/what-we-do/health-topics/communicable-diseases/hivaids/publications/2011/european-action-plan-for-hivaids-20122015).

104. European strategic action plan on antibiotic resistance. Copenhagen: WHO Regional Office for Europe; 2011 (EUR/RC61/14; http://www.euro.who.int/en/who-we-are/governance/regional-committee-for-europe/sixty-first-session/documentation/working-documents/wd14-european-strategic-action-plan-on-antibiotic-resistance).

105. WHO Regional Office for Europe, ECDC. Tuberculosis surveillance and monitoring in Europe 2012. Stockholm: European Centre for Disease Prevention and Control; 2012 (http://www.euro.who.int/en/health-topics/communicable-diseases/tuberculosis/publications/2012/tuberculosis-surveillance-and-monitoring-in-europe-2012).

106. WHO Regional Office for Europe, ECDC. Tuberculosis surveillance and monitoring in Europe 2013. Stockholm: European Centre for Disease Prevention and Control; 2012 (http://www.euro.who.int/en/health-topics/communicable-diseases/tuberculosis/publications/2013/tuberculosis-surveillance-and-monitoring-in-europe-2013).

107. WHO Regional Office for Europe, ECDC. HIV/AIDS surveillance in Europe 2011. Stockholm: European Centre for Disease Prevention and Control; 2012 (http://www.euro.who.int/en/what-we-do/health-topics/communicable-diseases/hivaids/publications/2012/hivaids-surveillance-in-europe-2011).

108. WHO Regional Office for Europe, ECDC. HIV/AIDS surveillance in Europe 2012. Stockholm: European Centre for Disease Prevention and Control; 2013 (http://www.euro.who.int/en/

health-topics/communicable-diseases/hivaids/publications/2013/hivaids-surveillance-in-europe-2012).

109. Best practices in prevention, control and care for drug-resistant tuberculosis. A resource for the continued implementation of the Consolidated Action Plan to Prevent and Combat Multidrug- and Extensively Drug-Resistant Tuberculosis in the WHO European Region, 2011–2015. Copenhagen: WHO Regional Office for Europe; 2013 (http://www.euro.who.int/en/health-topics/communicable-diseases/tuberculosis/publications/2013/best-practices-in-prevention,-control-and-care-for-drug-resistant-tuberculosis).

110. Revised guidance on HIV treatment and care published [website]. Copenhagen: WHO Regional Office for Europe; 2013 (http://www.euro.who.int/en/what-we-do/health-topics/communicable-diseases/hivaids/news/news/2012/2/revised-guidance-on-hiv-treatment-and-care-published).

111. HIV/AIDS country profiles [website]. Copenhagen: WHO Regional Office for Europe; 2013 (http://www.euro.who.int/en/what-we-do/health-topics/communicable-diseases/hivaids/country-work/hivaids-country-profiles).

112. Consolidated guidelines on the use of antiretroviral drugs for treating and preventing HIV infection. Recommendations for a public health approach. Geneva: World Health Organization; 2013 (http://www.who.int/hiv/pub/guidelines/arv2013/download/en/index.html).

113. Report of the 26th Meeting of the European Regional Certification Commission for Poliomyelitis Eradication. Copenhagen: WHO Regional Office for Europe; 2013 (http://www.euro.who.int/en/health-topics/communicable-diseases/poliomyelitis/publications/2013/report-of-the-26th-meeting-of-the-european-regional-certification-commission-for-poliomyelitis-eradication).

114. WHO EpiBrief and WHO EpiData [website]. Copenhagen: WHO Regional Office for Europe; 2013 (http://www.euro.who.int/en/what-we-do/health-topics/disease-prevention/vaccines-and-immunization/publications/who-epibrief-and-who-epidata).

115. Regional decline in measles with large rubella outbreaks in two countries: epidemiological overview for 2012 [website]. Copenhagen: WHO Regional Office for Europe; 2013 (http://www.euro.who.int/en/what-we-do/health-topics/communicable-diseases/measles-and-rubella/news/news/2013/05/regional-decline-in-measles-with-large-rubella-outbreaks-in-two-countries-epidemiological-overview-for-2012).

116. Progress report on measles and rubella elimination and the package for accelerated action to achieve elimination by 2015. Copenhagen: WHO Regional Office for Europe; 2013 (EUR/RC63/12; http://www.euro.who.int/en/who-we-are/governance/regional-committee-for-europe/sixty-third-session/working-documents/eurrc6312-progress-report-on-measles-and-rubella-elimination-and-the-package-for-accelerated-action).

117. Guide to tailoring immunization programmes (TIP). Copenhagen: WHO Regional Office for Europe; 2013 (http://www.euro.who.int/en/what-we-do/health-topics/disease-prevention/vaccines-and-immunization/publications/2013/guide-to-tailoring-immunization-programmes).

118. Guidelines for measles and rubella outbreak investigation and response in the WHO European Region. Copenhagen: WHO Regional Office for

Europe; 2013 (http://www.euro.who.int/en/health-topics/communicable-diseases/measles-and-rubella/publications/2013/guidelines-for-measles-and-rubella-outbreak-investigation-and-response-in-the-who-european-region).

119. European Immunization Week [website]. Copenhagen: WHO Regional Office for Europe; 2013 (http://www.euro.who.int/en/health-topics/disease-prevention/vaccines-and-immunization/european-immunization-week).

120. Immunization Resource Centre [website]. Copenhagen: WHO Regional Office for Europe; 2013 (http://www.euro.who.int/en/health-topics/disease-prevention/vaccines-and-immunization/vaccines-and-immunization/immunization-resource-centre).

121. Influenza [website]. Copenhagen: WHO Regional Office for Europe; 2013 (http://www.euro.who.int/en/health-topics/communicable-diseases/influenza).

122. Regional framework for surveillance and control of invasive mosquito vectors and re-emerging vector-borne diseases, 2014–2020. Copenhagen: WHO Regional Office for Europe; 2013 (http://www.euro.who.int/en/health-topics/communicable-diseases/vector-borne-and-parasitic-diseases/publications/2013/regional-framework-for-surveillance-and-control-of-invasive-mosquito-vectors-and-re-emerging-vector-borne-diseases,-20142020).

123. International Health Regulations [website]. Copenhagen: WHO Regional Office for Europe; 2013 (http://www.euro.who.int/ihr).

124. Disaster preparedness and response [website]. Copenhagen: WHO Regional Office for Europe; 2013 (http://www.euro.who.int/en/health-topics/emergencies/disaster-preparedness-and-response).

125. Assessment of health-system crisis preparedness: Israel. Copenhagen: WHO Regional Office for Europe; 2012 (http://www.euro.who.int/en/what-we-do/health-topics/emergencies/disaster-preparedness-and-response/publications/2012/assessment-of-health-system-crisis-preparedness-israel).

126. Strengthening health-system emergency preparedness. Toolkit for assessing health-system capacity for crisis management. Part 1. User manual. Copenhagen: WHO Regional Office for Europe; 2012 (http://www.euro.who.int/en/what-we-do/health-topics/emergencies/disaster-preparedness-and-response/publications/2012/strengthening-health-system-emergency-preparedness.-toolkit-for-assessing-health-system-capacity-for-crisis-management.-part-1.-user-manual).

127. Strengthening health-system emergency preparedness. Toolkit for assessing health-system capacity for crisis management. Part 2. Assessment form. Copenhagen: WHO Regional Office for Europe; 2012 (http://www.euro.who.int/en/what-we-do/health-topics/emergencies/disaster-preparedness-and-response/publications/2012/strengthening-health-system-emergency-preparedness.-toolkit-for-assessing-health-system-capacity-for-crisis-management.-part-2.-assessment-form).

128. Emergency Response Framework. Geneva: World Health Organization; 2013 (http://www.who.int/entity/hac/about/erf_.pdf).

129. Health planning for large public events [website]. Copenhagen: WHO Regional Office for Europe; 2013 (http://www.euro.who.int/en/what-we-do/health-topics/emergencies/disaster-preparedness-

and-response/activities/health-planning-for-large-public-events).

130. WHO/Europe influenza surveillance (EuroFlu.org) [website]. Copenhagen: WHO Regional Office for Europe; 2013 (http://www.euroflu.org).

131. Environment and health [website]. Copenhagen: WHO Regional Office for Europe; 2013 (http://www.euro.who.int/en/health-topics/environment-and-health).

132. Parma Declaration on Environment and Health. Copenhagen: WHO Regional Office for Europe; 2010 (http://www.euro.who.int/en/who-we-are/policy-documents/parma-declaration-on-environment-and-health).

133. Environment and health. Governance [website]. Copenhagen: WHO Regional Office for Europe; 2013 (http://www.euro.who.int/en/what-we-do/health-topics/environment-and-health/european-process-on-environment-and-health/governance).

134. Report of the European Environment and Health Ministerial Board to the WHO Regional Committee for Europe and the United Nations Economic Commission for Europe Committee on Environmental Policy. Copenhagen: WHO Regional Office for Europe; 2013 (EUR/RC63/10; http://www.euro.who.int/en/who-we-are/governance/regional-committee-for-europe/sixty-third-session/documentation/working-documents/eurrc6310-report-of-the-european-environment-and-health-ministerial-board-to-the-who-regional-committee-for-europe-and-the-united-nations-economic-commission-for-europe-committee-on-environmental-policy).

135. Report of the second (extraordinary) meeting of the European Environment and Health Task Force (EHTF). Copenhagen: WHO Regional Office for Europe; 2012 (http://www.euro.who.int/en/health-topics/environment-and-health/pages/european-environment-and-health-process-ehp/governance/european-environment-and-health-task-force-ehtf/report-of-the-second-extraordinary-meeting-of-the-european-environment-and-health-task-force-ehtf).

136. Workers' health: global plan of action. Geneva: World Health Organization; 2007 (http://www.who.int/occupational_health/publications/global_plan/en/index.html).

137. Protecting health from climate change: A seven-country initiative. Copenhagen: WHO Regional Office for Europe; 2013 (http://www.euro.who.int/en/health-topics/environment-and-health/Climate-change/publications/2013/protecting-health-from-climate-change-a-seven-country-initiative).

138. WHO evidence underpins new EU strategy on adapting to climate change [website]. Copenhagen: WHO Regional Office for Europe; 2013 (http://www.euro.who.int/en/what-we-do/health-topics/environment-and-health/Climate-change/news/news/2013/04/who-evidence-underpins-new-eu-strategy-on-adapting-to-climate-change).

139. Health aspects of air pollution and review of EU policies: the REVIHAAP and HRAPIE projects [website]. Copenhagen: WHO Regional Office for Europe; 2013 (http://www.euro.who.int/en/what-we-do/health-topics/environment-and-health/air-quality/activities/health-aspects-of-air-pollution-and-review-of-eu-policies-the-revihaap-and-hrapie-projects).

140. Health effects of particulate matter. Policy implications for countries in eastern Europe, Caucasus and central Asia. Copenhagen: WHO

Regional Office for Europe; 2013 (http://www.euro.who.int/en/what-we-do/health-topics/environment-and-health/air-quality/publications/2013/health-effects-of-particulate-matter.-policy-implications-for-countries-in-eastern-europe,-caucasus-and-central-asia).

141. Janssen NAH, Gerlofs-Nijland ME, Lanki T, Salonen RO, Cassee F, Hoek G et al. Health effects of black carbon. Copenhagen: WHO Regional Office for Europe; 2012 (http://www.euro.who.int/en/what-we-do/health-topics/environment-and-health/air-quality/publications/2012/health-effects-of-black-carbon).

142. Climate change and health: a tool to estimate health and adaptation costs. Copenhagen: WHO Regional Office for Europe; 2013 (http://www.euro.who.int/en/publications/abstracts/climate-change-and-health-a-tool-to-estimate-health-and-adaptation-costs).

143. Environmental health and economics: use of economic tools and methods in environmental health. Copenhagen: WHO Regional Office for Europe; 2013 (http://www.euro.who.int/en/health-topics/environment-and-health/health-impact-assessment/publications/2012/environmental-health-and-economics-use-of-economic-tools-and-methods-in-environmental-health).

144. Burden of disease from environmental noise. Quantification of healthy life years lost in Europe. Copenhagen: WHO Regional Office for Europe; 2011 (http://www.euro.who.int/en/what-we-do/health-topics/environment-and-health/noise/publications/2011/burden-of-disease-from-environmental-noise.-quantification-of-healthy-life-years-lost-in-europe).

145. WHO/Europe in Copenhagen moving to new premises [website]. Copenhagen: WHO Regional Office for Europe; 2013 (http://www.euro.who.int/en/what-we-do/health-topics/Health-systems/nursing-and-midwifery/news/news/2013/03/whoeurope-in-copenhagen-moving-to-new-premises).

146. WHO reform process: documents [website]. Geneva: World Health Organization; 2013 (http://www.who.int/about/who_reform/documents/en).

147. WHO reform. Copenhagen: WHO Regional Office for Europe; 2012 (EUR/RC62/14; http://www.euro.who.int/en/who-we-are/governance/regional-committee-for-europe/sixty-second-session/documentation/working-documents/eurrc6214-who-reform).

148. Draft proposed programme budget 2014–2015. Copenhagen: WHO Regional Office for Europe; 2012 (EUR/RC62/16; http://www.euro.who.int/en/who-we-are/governance/regional-committee-for-europe/sixty-second-session/documentation/working-documents/eurrc6216-draft-proposed-programme-budget-20142015).

149. The programme budget 2014–2015 – the perspective of the WHO Regional Office for Europe. Copenhagen: WHO Regional Office for Europe; 2012 (EUR/RC62/16 Add.1; http://www.euro.who.int/en/who-we-are/governance/regional-committee-for-europe/sixty-second-session/documentation/working-documents/eurrc6216-add.1-the-programme-budget-20142015-the-perspective-of-the-who-regional-office-for-europe).

150. Implementing the programme budget 2014–2015. Copenhagen: WHO Regional Office for Europe; 2013 (EUR/RC63/21; http://www.euro.who.int/en/who-we-are/governance/regional-committee-for-europe/sixty-third-session/working-documents/eurrc6321-implementing-the-programme-budget-20142015).

151. Implementing the programme budget 2014–2015. Copenhagen: WHO Regional Office for Europe; 2013 (EUR/RC63/21 Corr.1; http://www.euro.who.int/en/who-we-are/governance/regional-committee-for-europe/sixty-third-session/working-documents/eurrc6321-corr.1-implementing-the-programme-budget-20142015).

152. Governance reform in the WHO European Region. Copenhagen: WHO Regional Office for Europe; 2013 (EUR/RC63/16 Rev.1; http://www.euro.who.int/en/who-we-are/governance/regional-committee-for-europe/sixty-third-session/working-documents/eurrc6316-rev.1-governance-reform-in-the-who-european-region).

153. A review of the status of resolutions adopted by the Regional Committee during the past ten years (2003–2012), and recommendations for sunsetting and reporting requirements. Copenhagen: WHO Regional Office for Europe; 2013 (EUR/RC63/17 Rev.1; http://www.euro.who.int/en/about-us/governance/regional-committee-for-europe/archive/advance-copies-of-documents/eurrc6317-rev.1-a-review-of-the-status-of-resolutions-adopted-by-the-regional-committee-during-the-past-ten-years-20032012,-and-recommendations-for-sunsetting-and-reporting-requirements).

154. Report of the launch of WHO's financing dialogue. Copenhagen: WHO Regional Office for Europe; 2013 (EUR/RC63/19; http://www.euro.who.int/en/who-we-are/governance/regional-committee-for-europe/sixty-third-session/documentation/working-documents/eurrc6319-report-of-the-launch-of-whos-financing-dialogue).

155. Programme budget portal [website]. Geneva: World Health Organization; 2013 (https://extranet.who.int/programmebudget).

156. Stronger collaboration with the European Food Safety Authority [website]. Copenhagen: WHO Regional Office for Europe; 2012 (http://www.euro.who.int/en/who-we-are/partners/news/news/2012/07/stronger-collaboration-with-the-european-food-safety-authority).

157. WHO Representation to the European Union, Brussels, Belgium [website]. Copenhagen: WHO Regional Office for Europe; 2013 (http://www.euro.who.int/en/who-we-are/who-representation-to-the-european-union,-brussels,-belgium).

158. A country strategy for the WHO Regional Office for Europe 2012–2014. Copenhagen: WHO Regional Office for Europe; 2012 (EUR/RC62/13; http://www.euro.who.int/en/who-we-are/governance/regional-committee-for-europe/sixty-second-session/documentation/working-documents/eurrc6213-a-country-strategy-for-the-who-regional-office-for-europe-20122014).

159. WHO and Switzerland sign country cooperation strategy [website]. Copenhagen: WHO Regional Office for Europe; 2013 (http://www.euro.who.int/en/who-we-are/regional-director/news/news/2013/05/who-and-switzerland-sign-country-cooperation-strategy).

160. Publications [website]. Copenhagen: WHO Regional Office for Europe; 2013 (http://www.euro.who.int/en/publications).

161. European Health for All Database (HFA-DB) [online/offline database]. Copenhagen: WHO Regional Office for Europe; 2013 (http://www.euro.who.int/en/data-and-evidence/databases/european-health-for-all-database-hfa-db).

162. Media centre [website]. Copenhagen: WHO Regional Office for Europe; 2013 (http://www.euro.who.int/en/media-centre).

ANNEX: IMPLEMENTATION OF THE PROGRAMME BUDGET FOR 2012–2013

Tables 1 and 2 and Fig. 1 show the progress of the WHO Regional Office for Europe in implementing the programme budget for 2012–2013 that was approved by the World Health Assembly. Overall, 97% of the approved budget was implemented.

TABLE 1. Size and implementation of the programme budget (PB) of the WHO Regional Office for Europe by budget segment (US$ millions), 31 December 2013

Segment	PB		Funds			Implementation as % of:		
	Approved	Allocated	Available	Implemented	Available as % of approved PB	Approved PB	Allocated PB	Funds available
Base	192	213	198	185	103	97	87	93
Special programmes and collaborative arrangements	10	29	21	19	204	186	67	91
Outbreak and crisis response	11	11	1	1	13	12	12	93
Total	213	253	221	206	104	97	81	93

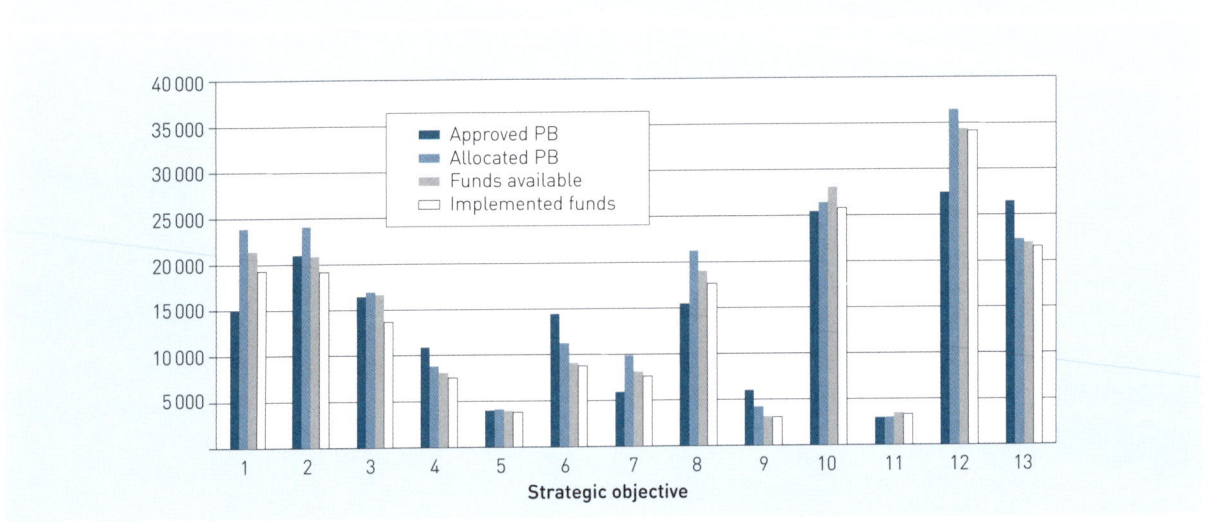

FIG. 1. Base segment of the Regional Office PB (US$ thousands), 31 December 2013

TABLE 2. Base segment of the Regional Office PB by strategic objective (SO) (US$ thousands), 31 December 2013

SO	PB		Funds			Implementation as % of:		
	Approved	Allocated	Available	Implemented	Available as % of approved PB	Approved PB	Allocated PB	Funds available
1	15 000	23 931	21 442	19 289	143	129	81	90
2	21 000	24 135	20 857	19 162	99	91	79	92
3	16 500	16 995	16 681	13 703	101	83	81	82
4	10 900	8 845	8 102	7 547	74	69	85	93
5	4 000	4 166	3 959	3 789	99	95	91	96
6	14 500	11 339	9 103	8 758	63	60	77	96
7	5 900	9 907	8 114	7 584	138	129	77	93
8	15 500	21 267	19 032	17 656	123	114	83	93
9	6 000	4 263	3 136	3 105	52	52	73	99
10	25 500	26 464	28 078	25 794	110	101	97	92
11	3 000	3 030	3 509	3 313	117	110	109	94
12	27 500	36 509	34 393	34 146	125	124	94	99
13	26 500	22 408	22 030	21 548	83	81	96	98
Total	191 800	213 259	198 437	185 395	103	97	87	93